ERGONOMICS AND CUMULATIVE TRAUMA DISORDERS

A Handbook for Occupational Therapists

Ergonomics and Cumulative Trauma Disorders

A Handbook for Occupational Therapists

Denise Kenny Claiborne, M.S., OTR, CHT
Nancy J. Powell, Ph.D., FAOTA
Kathleen Reynolds-Lynch, M.S., OTR, FAOTA

SINGULAR PUBLISHING GROUP, INC.
SAN DIEGO • LONDON

Singular Publishing Group, Inc.
401 West A Street, Suite 325
San Diego, California 92101-7904

Singular Publishing Ltd.
19 Compton Terrace
London N1 2UN, UK

Singular Publishing Group, Inc., publishes textbooks, clinical manuals, clinical reference books, journals, videos, and multimedia materials on speech-language pathology, audiology, otorhinolaryngology, special education, early childhood, aging, occupational therapy, physical therapy, rehabilitation, counseling, mental health and voice. For your convenience, our entire catalog can be accessed on our webside at *http://www.singpub.com.* Our mission to provide you with materials to meet the daily challenges of the ever-changing health care/educational environment will remain on course if we are in touch with you. In that spirit, we welcome your feedback on our products. Please telephone (**1-800-521-8545**), fax (**1-800-774-8398**), or e-mail (*singpub@singpub.com*) your comments and requests to us.

Typeset in 11/13 Bookman Light by Thompson Type
Printed in the United States of America by McNaughton and Gunn

Library of Congress Cataloging-in-Publication Data

Claiborne, Denise Kenny.
   Ergonomics and cumulative trauma disorders : a handbook for occupational therapists / Denise Kenny Claiborne, Nancy J. Powell, Kathleeen Reynolds-Lynch.
      p.   cm.
   Includes bibliographical references.
   ISBN 0-7693-0024-3 (soft cover : alk. paper)
   1. Overuse injuries—Prevention—Handbooks, manuals, etc.   2. Human engineering—Handbooks, manuals, etc.   3. Occupational therapy services—Handbooks, manuals, etc.   I. Powell, Nancy J.
II. Reynolds-Lynch, Kathleen.   III. Title.
   [DNLM: 1. Cumulative Trauma Disorders—prevention & control.   2. Human Engineering.
3. Occupational Diseases—prevention & control.   4. Arm Injuries—prevention & control.
5. Occupational Therapy.   WE 175 C585e 1999]
RD97.6.C56   1999
617.1—dc21
DNLM/DLC
for Library of Congress   98-50553
                                                                                                                              CIP

Contents

APPENDIXES

Preface

The purpose of this manual is to aid occupational therapists and students who are interested in providing ergonomic services. This manual is written at the introductory level. It is designed to be used in two ways, as an *instructional tool* and as a *reference book*. As an instructional tool, it provides occupational therapists with an introduction to ergonomics and cumulative trauma disorders. Following review of this manual, the occupational therapist should have beginning knowledge in the following areas:

- Ergonomics
- Cumulative trauma disorders including causes, structures involved, and types
- Cumulative trauma prevention programs
- The theoretical base and role of the occupational therapist in ergonomics
- General practice guidelines for occupational therapists in ergonomics
- Specific guidelines for providing occupational therapy-related ergonomic services including risk analysis, employer and employee education sessions, specialized work assessments, individual worker education sessions, and job coaching
- Brief review of cumulative trauma disorders and computer users

This manual is also designed to be used as a reference book. An occupational therapist providing ergonomic services may refer to this manual for further information on specific ergonomic topics.

The emphasis of this manual is ergonomics and upper extremity cumulative trauma disorders related to industrial work. Back injuries are out of the scope of this book. A brief section and related references are included on office ergonomics. A thorough review of this topic is out of the scope of this book.

In addition to this manual, an occupational therapist may need training in ergonomics, including review of the literature and attendance at various ergonomic-related conferences and courses. Additional training is needed to provide a greater knowledge base and skill level prior to providing these services. This manual includes suggested resources for broadening the therapist's knowledge base in ergonomics and cumulative trauma disorders. These resources are listed in Appendix A and include books, journals, associations, and Internet Web sites.

Acknowledgments

Our sincere appreciation is extended to our friends, family, coworkers, and colleagues who offered assistance with this manual. Karen Williams provided support, guidance, and suggestions throughout preparation of this book. Frank Stein reviewed this text and offered helpful suggestions. We would also like to thank the staff at Singular Publishing Group, especially Candice Janco, for their support and guidance during the book production. A special thanks to George Claiborne for his support, suggestions, and unending computer operation guidance.

CHAPTER I

Ergonomics

Ergonomics is defined as the "scientific study of the relationship between man, work and the working environment. It incorporates the use of physiological and physical engineering principles to make motion, function and work safe and efficient" (Isernhagen, 1988, p. 54). Ergonomics is designed to do the following (Isernhagen, Hart, & Matheson, 1998):

1. Increase group and individual productivity

2. Improve worker safety

3. Decrease lost time due to illness or injury

Poorly designed workplaces create an unsafe work system. Ergonomics "provides solutions to design problems involving human integration with a system" (Imker, 1993, p. 8). The benefits of ergonomics include increasing worker productivity while containing costs associated with work-related injuries (Devlin, 1993).

Ergonomics is both a science and an art. It requires both scientific knowledge and artistic ability/experience. The artistic ability is necessary because of the significant variability among humans. Humans are not machines. Everyone has an individual response to his or her work and work environment. The scientific basis of ergonomics relies on engineering, biomechanics, psychology, physiology, and metabolism (Isernhagen et al., 1998).

Employers are required by the Occupational Safety and Health Act (1970) to maintain a safe workplace that is free from recognized hazards (Kenny, Powell, & Reynolds-Lynch, 1995). The Occupational Safety and Health Administration (OSHA) uses this act to address ergonomic issues. OSHA developed ergonomic meat-packing guidelines in 1991 to assist employers in that industry with reducing and managing work-related injuries (Weber & Karen, 1998). OSHA is presently redirecting its focus from high-hazard industrial workplaces to all workplaces (Moore, 1990). OSHA is also focusing on cumulative trauma disorders. OSHA is in the process of creating proposed ergonomic rules for all workplaces. A draft of these proposed standards was released March 20, 1995 (Weber & Karen, 1998). These rules are predicted to be similar to the ergonomic meat-packing guidelines but expanded to address all workplaces. Employers are expected to seek assistance from both medical and engineering professionals to comply with OSHA's ergonomic rules.

Congress is currently targeting OSHA for deregulation. This could limit OSHA's power and authority needed to enforce the ergonomic standards. OSHA's standards may therefore be changed from standards to guidelines (Weber & Karen, 1998).

The National Institute of Occupational Safety and Health (NIOSH) is the agency responsible for research studies dealing with safety and health problems. NIOSH is actively researching CTDs. They have proposed standards : "Control of Work Related CTDs, Part 1: Upper Extremities." These standards were released in March 1996 (ANSI, 1996).

Occupational therapists are uniquely qualified to provide specialized ergonomic services to assist employers with OSHA compliance. Occupational therapists have a medical background as well as a holistic approach for problem (risk) identification and ergonomic risk resolution. The theoretical role of the occupational therapist and ergonomics as well as a description of occupational therapy ergonomic practice guidelines are included in Chapter 4 of this manual.

CHAPTER 2

Cumulative Trauma Disorders

A major emphasis of ergonomics is the reduction of cumulative trauma disorders (CTDs). Cumulative trauma disorders are musculoskeletal conditions that develop gradually as a result of repeated microtrauma. *Cumulative* is defined as repeated stress on a particular body part over a period of time. *Trauma* is defined as injury to the body from an outside source (Isernhagen, S. J., 1998). These disorders are also referred to as repetitive strain disorders, overuse syndromes, work-related musculoskeletal disorders, and repetitive motion disorders (Weber & Karen, 1998). The term *CTD* is used in this manual.

These disorders are typically considered to be work related, as they are more prevalent among working people than the general population (Putz-Anderson, 1988). However, these injuries can also result from non–work-related tasks (e.g., golf, tennis, and video games). This manual focuses on work-related upper extremity CTDs. The primary emphasis of this manual is industrial-related CTDs. However, a brief review of computer-related CTDs is included.

INCIDENCE

The incidence of CTDs is reaching epidemic proportions. It has been estimated that almost 19 million U.S. workers per year are affected with CTDs, costing industry nearly $100 billion annually (LaBar, 1991). The occupational incidence rates for 1997 were 62.3 percent (Isernhagen, D., 1998). Some causes for the increased incidence of CTDs include specialization, minimal variability of muscle groups used, incentive-driven production programs, and voluntary overtime (Kenny et al., 1995; Weber & Karen, 1998). The highest percentage of work-related CTDs occurs in the manufacturing sector (e.g., assembly line work) (Keller, Corbett, & Nichols, 1998). The incidence of CTDs will continue to grow unless ergonomic programs are initiated to help reduce and manage these disorders.

CAUSATIVE FACTORS

Armstrong (1994) described two groups of CTD causative factors, occupational and nonoccupational. Nonoccupational factors may include arthritis, acute trauma, endocrine disease, age, gender, wrist size or shape, pregnancy, and oral contraceptives. Nonoccupational factors may also include recreational activities and vocational interests. Occupational factors related to CTDs may include static muscle contractions, repetition, force, awkward postures, vibration, cold, and localized contact pressure (Armstrong, 1994). This manual describes each of the occupational factors in detail. The occupational factors are defined and methods for identifying and reducing these factors at the worksite are outlined in the risk analysis section in Chapter 5 of this manual.

CONTROVERSY

Recently there has been increased debate over CTD causes. Some current data suggest predisposing genetic factors may explain why some workers get CTDs and others do not, even though they are doing the same job (Beattie, 1995). Several studies support and refute the relationship between CTDs and ergonomic risks. The University of Michigan Center for Ergonomics researchers have documented that work activities requiring high force and high repetition result in a significantly higher incidence of CTDs. Another study

(Nathan, 1990) disputed these findings and did not find a significant relationship between the intensity of work and the development of CTDs (Werner, 1997).

The factors involved with CTD cause and effect will be defined by litigation. The debate between the medical and legal professions to determine if CTDs are related to ergonomic stressors continues (Isernhagen et al., 1998). Specific CTD diagnosis (particularly carpal tunnel syndrome and thoracic outlet syndrome) and ergonomic risk factors (especially repetition) are being looked at closely. Further studies are needed.

ANATOMICAL STRUCTURES AFFECTED BY CTDs

Cumulative trauma disorders develop in soft tissues. Muscles, tendons, blood vessels, and nerves are primarily affected.

- Muscles are the force producing structures of the body. Muscles contract and elicit exertions and movements around joints. Muscles can be injured when their fibers are strained, irritated, or torn apart. Muscles can also be injured from a severe blow or crush resulting in broken blood vessels. Interrupted muscular blood and/ or nerve supply can result in muscle atrophy (Putz-Anderson, 1988). Common CTDs associated with muscles include fatigue, myositis, and myofascial pain (Armstrong, 1994).

- Tendons are the load-bearing structures that connect muscle to bone. Tendons are encased in synovial sheaths that secrete fluid. This fluid nourishes the tendon and lubricates the tendon for easy gliding. Overuse may decrease the amount of synovial fluid and cause friction between the tendon and its sheath. This could result in inflammation of the tendons and synovial sheaths (Putz-Anderson, 1988). Examples of CTDs affecting tendons include synovitis, tenosynovitis, bursitis, stenosing tenosynovitis, De Quervain's, and epicondylitis (Armstrong, 1994).

- Blood vessels supply nourishment to muscles and tendons and remove waste from these structures. CTDs affecting blood vessels can result in oxygen and nutrient deprivation to surrounding tissues. Blood vessels may be injured when exposed to pressure or compression from a sharp surface or surrounding structures. Common types of CTDs affecting blood vessels include thoracic outlet syndrome and Raynaud's phenomenon (Putz-Anderson, 1988).

- Nerves are the communication network of the body. CTDs may result in motor and sensory nerve disturbances. Nerves may be injured when exposed to pressure or compression from sharp surfaces, nearby bones, ligaments, and tendons (Putz-Anderson, 1988). Nerve-related CTDs include thoracic outlet syndrome, cubital tunnel syndrome, digital neuritis, and carpal tunnel syndrome (Armstrong, 1994).

TYPES OF UPPER EXTREMITY CTDs

The three types of CTDs are tendon disorders, nerve disorders, and neurovascular disorders.

Tendon Disorders

The symptoms of CTDs affecting tendons include dull aching sensation over the tendon, discomfort with specific movements, and tenderness to touch. Tendon disorders typically occur at the tendon–muscle juncture near joints where they rub adjacent structures (Putz-Anderson, 1988). The following is a list and brief description of common tendon-related CTDs.

1. *Tendinitis* is an inflamed unsheathed tendon that may become frayed or torn apart when repeatedly exerted and tensed. The tendon may become thickened, bumpy, and irregular. Tendons without sufficient rest and recovery time may become permanently weakened (Putz-Anderson, 1988).

2. *Tenosynovitis* is an inflammation of the tendon and its surrounding synovial sheath. Extreme repetition stimulates the sheath to secrete excessive fluid that accumulates, causing the sheath to become swollen and painful. The tendon surface may become thickened or frayed and adhesions may form. Extensor tendons, particularly along the radial border of the forearm, are most commonly affected (Pheasant, 1991).

3. *Stenosing tenosynovitis (trigger finger)* is a form of tenosynovitis in which the tendon movement within the sheath is limited. The swollen sheath constricts the tendon and limits tendon gliding (Pheasant, 1991).

4. *De Quervain's disease ("washerwoman's sprain")* is a form of tenosynovitis affecting the first dorsal (extensor) compartment. The extensor pollicis brevis and abductor pollicis longus are involved (Kirkpatrick, 1990).

5. *Lateral epicondylitis ("tennis elbow")* is a form of tendinitis affecting the wrist and digit extensors where they originate at the lateral epicondyle of the humerus. Overuse of these muscles may result in microtears where the tendon originates at the bone (Pheasant, 1991).

6. *Medial epicondylitis ("golfer's elbow")* is another form of tendinitis affecting the wrist and digit flexors where they originate at the medial epicondyle of the elbow (Pheasant, 1991).

7. *Rotator cuff tendinitis* is also known as supraspinatous tendinitis, subdeltoid bursitis, subacromial bursitis, and partial tear of rotator cuff. The four rotator cuff tendons provide the shoulder with mobility and stability. These tendons internally and externally rotate and abduct the arm. Repeated overhead motions result in wear and tear of the tendons as they pass between the humerus and acromion process (Putz-Anderson, 1988).

Nerve Disorders

Common symptoms of CTDs affecting nerves include pain and paresthesia following the involved nerve's distribution pattern distal to the sight of injury. Nocturnal burning pain is also frequently reported (Baxter-Petralia, 1990). Nerve-related CTDs occur when nerves are exposed to sustained or repeated pressure from internal structures or external hard, sharp edges (Putz-Anderson, 1988). The following is a list and brief description of common nerve-related CTDs.

1. *Carpal tunnel syndrome (CTS)* is the result of median nerve compression within the carpal tunnel. The carpal tunnel is composed of eight irregular shaped carpal bones covered by the tough fibrous flexor retinaculum. The tunnel contains the finger flexor tendons and the median nerve. The median nerve innervates most of the palm, thumb, index finger, middle finger, and radial border of the ring finger (Pheasant, 1991). Finger flexor tendon sheaths that become swollen may impinge

on the median nerve within the cramped carpal tunnel. The symptoms of carpal tunnel syndrome include numbness, tingling, and pain in the distal distribution of the median nerve. These symptoms commonly wake patients during the night. In advanced cases, the symptoms may persist during the day, the person may drop objects frequently owing to decreased sensation, and thenar muscle atrophy is commonly observed (Putz-Anderson, 1988).

2. *Cubital tunnel syndrome* is compression of the ulnar nerve as it passes through a ligamentous tunnel posterior to the medial epicondyle of the humerus. Symptoms of this disorder include pain, tingling sensation, and numbness along the medial side of the forearm to the little finger (Pheasant, 1991).

3. *Guyon's Canal* is compression of the ulnar nerve at the wrist. The symptoms may include weakness of the interosseous muscles of the hand (Pheasant, 1991).

Neurovascular Disorders

Both nerves and the adjacent blood vessels are affected by neurovascular CTDs. Common symptoms of neurovascular CTDs include numbness, blanched skin, and weakened pulse (Putz-Anderson, 1988). Common neurovascular CTDs and a brief description are listed below.

1. *Thoracic outlet syndrome (TOS)* is a neurovascular compression at the shoulder. The brachial plexus can be compressed within the thoracic outlet. The thoracic outlet is composed of the anterior scalene muscle, medial scalene muscle, clavicle, and first rib. There may be congenital or structural predisposing risk factors related to this syndrome (Whitenack, Hunter, Jaeger, & Read, 1990). Activities and postures of the upper extremity can impede circulation by putting pressure on the blood vessels within the thoracic outlet. Decreased circulation results in oxygen and nutrient deprivation to surrounding tendons, ligaments, and muscles. Muscle recovery and activity duration are slowed and limited (Putz-Anderson, 1988). The common symptoms of TOS include pain, paresthesias, and weakness in the involved arm. The symptoms often follow the ulnar nerve distribution in the hand (little finger and ulnar border of the ring finger). There may be sensory overlaps (Whitenack et al., 1990).

2. *Raynaud's phenomenon (vibration syndrome and white finger)* is characterized by frequent finger blanching as a result of constriction of the digital arteries. Vasospasms in the fingers may be triggered by cold temperatures. Causative factors may include prolonged gripping and use of vibratory tools. The symptoms include frequent digit numbness and tingling; pale, ashen, and cold skin; and loss of sensation and hand control (Putz-Anderson, 1988).

CHARACTERISTICS OF CTDs

The common symptoms of CTDs include pain, tenderness, weakness, swelling, and numbness. Kroemer (1989) identified *three stages of CTDs.*

■ The *first stage* is characterized by aches and fatigue occurring during work hours only. There is no change in work performance. The disorder is reversible at this point.

■ The *second stage* is characterized by symptoms that begin early in the work shift and do not resolve over night. At this point, work capacity is reduced.

■ The *third stage* is characterized by symptoms that persist even at rest. The worker has difficulty performing even light tasks.

Ergonomics has the greatest impact on stage one CTDs. Typically CTDs at stage one can be resolved with ergonomic intervention. A combination of medical attention and ergonomics is needed at advanced stages.

CHAPTER 3

Cumulative Trauma Disorder Prevention Programs

TRADITIONAL PROGRAMS

In the past, health promotion and injury prevention services were available primarily in the community (e.g., hospitals and clinics) (Kenny et al., 1995). When workers were injured at the worksite, they were typically sent out for medical care and returned to work when fully recovered from the injury. Typically, if injured workers did not fully recover from an injury, they were unable to return to work. Very few accommodations were made to assist with returning injured workers to work, and little effort was made to identify the causes of the injury and resolve work-related risks. Fully recovered workers often returned to the same positions on which they were injured, and their symptoms were often reaggravated. Reinjured workers were once again referred out for medical care. Chong (1993) referred to this recurrent pattern as the "worker's compensation loop."

PRESENT PROGRAMS

The current trend is the transfer of health promotion and injury prevention services from the community to the work site where many injuries occur. There are many benefits to having work-site health promotion and injury prevention programs, including health and cost benefits. All the studies Pelletier (1993) reviewed on the health and cost benefits of work-site injury prevention programs revealed positive results. Benefits identified were decreased absenteeism, enhanced productivity, improved company public image, assistance with attracting and retaining key personnel, and a greater allegiance to the company by employees (Pelletier, 1993).

When workers are injured at the work site, they are often referred to the company medical department. Injured workers receive immediate medical care at the work site. The staff of the company medical department may include physicians, nurses, occupational therapists, and physical therapists. Occasionally the injured workers are referred out for specialized medical care. Frequently workers continue working with restrictions that are dependent on the extent of their injuries (e.g., one-handed work, no overhead lifting, and no air-tool use).

The incidences of cumulative trauma disorders (CTDs) and their associated costs are steadily rising. Companies are beginning to set up on-site injury prevention and health promotion programs to decrease the number of CTDs and related costs. Reasons for increased emphasis on injury prevention and health promotion at the work site include the following:

■ Key negotiating point in union and labor contracts

■ Americans with Disabilities Act (ADA) legal considerations

■ Proposed OSHA ergonomic standards

■ Emphasis by managed health care systems

Efforts are being made to identify job risks and ergonomically eliminate these risks. The application of an ergonomics program can help to stop the worker's compensation loop (Chong, 1993). Most employers are interested in reducing injuries through health promotion and injury prevention programs, but they need help.

A TEAM APPROACH TO ERGONOMICS

Few fields are more interdisciplinary than ergonomics. "Designing work and living environments to meet human needs requires the combined knowledge of disciplines as diverse as healthcare, engineering, psychology and computer science" (Framoze, 1994, p. 37). A multidisciplinary ergonomic team approach is most effective with solving complex workplace problems. This approach pulls together knowledge from various disciplines. Professionals involved with ergonomics include engineers, safety engineers, organizational psychiatrists, industrial hygienists, exercise physiologists, rehabilitation engineers, occupational therapists, physical therapists, nurses, physicians, and physician's assistants (Rice & Jacobs, 1993; Butler, 1998). The diverse group of professionals providing ergonomic services must be aware of their professional limitations and utilize the expertise of other professions (Framoze, 1994). No one profession has all the skills and expertise needed to address the multiple factors of CTDs and ergonomics.

A comprehensive ergonomic program requires input and open communication among professionals from a variety of disciplines. Scheduled team meetings are recommended (perhaps quarterly). Outcomes are more successful when all parties are informed. Lack of communication can lead to adversarial relationships among team members (Butler, 1998).

Representative workers should be part of the ergonomic team. They are helpful with problem identification and ergonomic design (Isernhagen et al., 1998). No one knows the jobs better than the workers performing them. Involving workers will also assist with achieving their commitment to the ongoing ergonomic process. Some companies offer incentive programs for encouraging worker commitment. An example of an incentive program is offering workers gift certificates for ergonomic ideas. These ideas can be voted on at the ergonomic team meetings.

ERGONOMIC CERTIFICATION

Many professions are considering offering credentials in a subspecialty of ergonomics. Certification is offered by the Board of Certification in Professional Ergonomics (BCPE). A pilot certification exam was held May 16, 1998. The Certified Professional Ergonomist (CPE) designation is for professionals with a master's degree in human factors or ergonomics who practice ergonomics full time (Rice, 1998).

The Certified Ergonomics Associate (CEA) credentials are designated for professionals with a strong background in ergonomics, but for whom ergonomics is not their primary job. This credentialing is for professionals such as health professionals, industrial hygienists, safety professionals, and engineering and design professionals. Since most occupational therapists are not interested in pursuing a master's degree in ergonomics or human factors, the CEA credentials are perfect.

Rice (1998) identified the CEA credentialing requirements, which are listed as follows:

- Bachelor's or associate's degree
- 200 contact hours in ergonomics (training and instruction)
- Two years on-the-job ergonomic experience
- Passing score on the CEA exam

Occupational therapists who practice within the field of ergonomics typically focus on the prevention of musculoskeletal disorders. That is the primary emphasis of this book. Rice (1998) warns therapists interested in pursuing the CEA designation that they will need to supplement their ergonomic knowledge. The certification exam covers all areas of ergonomics, including cognitive, psychological, and physical components. For more information, BCPE contact information is listed in Appendix A of this book.

The Ergonomic Rehabilitation Society is investigating offering credentials to health ergonomists. The American Occupational Therapy Association special interest section in work programs is also considering credential programs for occupational therapists in ergonomics (Rice & Jacobs, 1993).

CHAPTER 4

Ergonomics and the Occupational Therapist

HISTORICAL BACKGROUND

Occupational therapists providing ergonomic services typically have a background in hand therapy, work hardening, and/or industrial rehabilitation. The occupational therapist in a work hardening (industrial rehabilitation) setting focuses on improving an injured worker's level of functioning specifically for return to work. The skills and treatment techniques the occupational therapist uses to treat industrial injuries in the clinic are easily applied to the work site.

The occupational therapist's background in work hardening provides skills and expertise in treating patients with industrial injuries and fosters communication and rapport with employers. This communication with employers leads to occupational therapists providing work-site ergonomic services. Through ergonomics, the occupational therapist assists with injury prevention and early return to work following an injury. The occupational therapy profession has a long history of involvement with industrial rehabilitation.

Occupational therapists' involvement in industrial rehabilitation can be traced back to the early 1900s. At that time occupational therapists were actively involved in developing industrial therapy programs in mental hospitals (Matheson, Ogden, Violette, & Schultz, 1985). In the 1920s, the World War I era, occupational therapists began offering vocational education and rehabilitative services to soldiers to help them achieve functional levels for employment. In the 1930s, occupational therapists expanded their focus to orthopedic problems and industrial accident patients (Taylor, 1993). The mechanization of American industry resulted in an increase in industrial accidents and therefore an increased need for occupational therapist intervention. Within the hospital, occupational therapists identified various jobs for the patients and coordinated patient work assignments based on the patients' aptitudes, interests, experiences, and therapeutic goals (Matheson et al., 1985).

In the 1940s, the World War II era, a work-evaluation program was developed at the Rochester Rehabilitation Center in New York. This program reconditioned people for return to work and supplied information for vocational goals. During the mid-1940s through the 1950s, occupational therapists established curative workshops. The goal of these workshops was to restore the patient to as normal function as possible, with return to work as the ultimate goal. In the late 1950s and 1960s, occupational therapists began to emphasize the medical model and their role in physical rehabilitation centers (Matheson, et al., 1985). The focus shifted away from industrial injury to increasing patients' independence in school, home, and community (Taylor, 1993).

Occupational therapists shifted their focus back to industry in the 1980s. Matheson and colleagues (1985) urged occupational therapists to apply their professional skills to the needs of modern industry. Occupational therapists transitioned from hospitals and schools to work-related services. Work hardening and ergonomics came to the forefront of occupational therapy in the 1980s. Reasons for the increased involvement of occupational therapy in this area include the increased number of industrial injury cases, increased worker's compensation costs, regulatory agency guidelines, and related legislation (e.g., the Americans with Disabilities Act). The American Occupational Therapy Association established its commitment to work programs through the establishment of a work program special interest section in 1986 (Jacobs, 1993).

Industrial rehabilitation is one of the fastest growing rehabilitation areas. In the 1990s, occupational therapists are redefining their services to business and industry. The areas of injury prevention and worker education are receiving increased emphasis. Automation may be the reason why occupational therapy emphasis on injury prevention and education has increased. Automation has resulted in a decrease in heavy lifting jobs with an increase in upper extremity intense jobs such as transcription work on a computer. These upper extremity intense jobs have led to the increased incidence of CTDs and demand for services to reduce and eliminate them. Occupational therapists have seen an increase in the number of patients they are treating with a history of CTDs. They are also being asked to provide ergonomic services at the work site to assist with reducing and eliminating these injuries. Another reason for increased occupational therapy involvement in injury prevention is the aging work force whose members are more vulnerable to CTDs and are interested in wellness and health promotion (Taylor, 1993).

THEORETICAL BASE

Occupational therapists are uniquely qualified to provide ergonomic services to business and industry. Not only have occupational therapists been involved in treating industrial injuries since the early 1900s, but occupational therapists have a theoretical base related to work. "Work is at the heart of the philosophy and practice of occupational therapy. In its broadest sense, work, as a productive activity, is the concern in almost all therapy" (Jacobs, 1985). The field of occupational therapy rests on the understanding that humans need activity and mastery over the environment. They will seek assistance in achieving optimum performance. Illness is believed to interfere with self-actualization. An injury or disability may interfere with a person's ability to work. The occupational therapist works to restore a person's ability to work (Mayer & Gatchel, 1988).

The major focus of occupational therapy is to increase independence in the performance areas of self-care, work, and leisure (Dutton, 1993). Independence in occupational performance is a goal of occupational therapy (Trombly, 1989). This goal is very similar to the goal of ergonomics, which is optimizing human performance and maximizing efficiency (Framoze, 1994).

Occupational therapists have a holistic approach focusing on the total person in relation to society and the world (Johnson, 1993). Industrial injuries are a complex problem and require a holistic approach. Occupational therapists have the ability to deal with physical and psychosocial issues (Mayer & Gatchel, 1988). For example, an occupational therapist will be able to recognize whether psychosocial or physical issues are the primary limiting factor for return to work following an injury.

Frame of Reference

The rehabilitative approach is the main frame of reference for occupational therapists providing ergonomic services (Trombly, 1989). However, other frames of reference (e.g., biomechanical and psychosocial approaches) may be used depending on the case.

The rehabilitative approach aims at increasing independence after an injury or disability. This approach assists with the identification of ways to compensate for a loss with adaptive techniques (e.g., alternating hands when performing a job task) and adaptive equipment (e.g., gloves and tool balancers). An example of the rehabilitative frame of reference using ergonomics is as follows:

> Ms. Jones is a 35-year-old women with a diagnosis of bilateral carpal tunnel syndrome. Her job title is billing clerk at a physician's office. The occupational therapist completed a job analysis through observation of the worker performing job duties and an interview with Ms. Jones and her supervisor. The job stresses and ergonomic risks identified include reported increased symptoms and decreased ability to type on a computer for

prolonged periods and to use a stapler. Through job coaching, Ms. Jones was instructed in *adaptive work techniques,* including maintaining a neutral wrist position while performing typing tasks and alternating typing tasks with other work tasks (e.g., writing, opening mail, and filing). *Adaptive equipment* recommended for Ms. Jones included computer wrist rests and an electric stapler. Using the adaptive techniques and equipment, Ms. Jones is able to perform job tasks *independently.*

Dutton (1993) identified the assumptions of this frame of reference. These assumptions are paraphrased as follows:

1. Independence is regained through compensation.
2. Motivation is influenced by lifelong values and the environment.
3. Minimal emotional and cognitive skills are needed to be independent.
4. Clinical reasoning should take a top-down approach.

Clinical reasoning is a concept that links practice with theory. Clinical reasoning takes a deductive reasoning approach. The five steps in the top-down hierarchy are listed as follows (Dutton, 1993):

1. Identify environmental demands (e.g., job analysis).
2. Identify current functional capability (e.g., on-site functional capacity evaluations).
3. Identify task demands that patients cannot perform (e.g., risk analysis and specialized work assessments).
4. Employ the rehabilitative frame of reference using compensatory methods and adaptive devices (e.g., built-up tool handles).
5. Identify specific modalities (e.g., one-handed technique).

Within this frame of reference, occupational therapists identify abilities and limits through observation and interview. The occupational therapist determines if the task can be safely and effectively accomplished (Trombly, 1989). An example of an ergonomic assessment completed through interview and observation is a job analysis. In a job analysis, an occupational therapist observes the worker performing a job task and then interviews the worker and his or her supervisor to identify job requirements.

Following identification of limits through assessment, the occupational therapist chooses treatment techniques to eliminate or improve the limiting factors (Trombly, 1989). For example, a small worker performing a job that requires repetitive above-shoulder-level reaching develops a case of rotator cuff tendinitis and cannot perform her job duties. To eliminate the limiting factor/risk of decreased tolerance for repetitive above-shoulder-level reaching, the occupational therapist recommends either that the part be lowered or that the worker stand on a platform to eliminate above-shoulder-level reaching. If the limiting factor cannot be eliminated or improved, the occupational therapist teaches adaptive ways of doing the task. For this example, the occupational therapist can teach the client to alternate upper extremities when reaching for the part.

ROLE OF THE OCCUPATIONAL THERAPIST

The role of the occupational therapist has expanded to meet the health care needs of business and industry. In this nontraditional community setting, occupational therapists are using the same skills they used to increase independence in home and school settings (Taylor, 1993) to increase independence and reduce CTD risks at the worksite. Occupational therapists' extensive training in observation, activity analysis, and adaptive methods uniquely prepares them for the field of ergonomics.

Observation is a preferred evaluation technique. The occupational therapist uses observation to detect unsafe methods and identify underlying reasons a task cannot be performed (Trombly, 1989). These observation skills are very useful when applied to the work setting. Through observation, occupational therapists can identify ergonomic risks, unsafe work methods, and reasons why a worker is having difficulty performing job tasks. An example of an ergonomic service that relies heavily on observation skills is a risk analysis. Through observation of a worker performing job duties, the occupational therapist can identify ergonomic risks. Specific guidelines for completing a risk analysis are included in Chapter 5, the risk analysis section of this manual.

"Activity analysis is one of the key process skills of the occupational therapist by which activities are closely examined to determine their components and what level of capability is demanded to enable a person to do the activity" (Trombly, 1989, p. 305). A specialized activity analysis is a job analysis. A job analysis identifies the components of a job and the physical demands of the job. Comparison between a job analysis and a worker's capabilities determines whether the worker will be able to do the job independently, with adaptation, or not at all. Guidelines for completing a job analysis are included in Chapter 5 of this manual.

The occupational therapists' skills in adapting tasks and methods can be directly applied to the work site. If there is a discrepancy between the job demands, as identified through a job analysis, and the physical capabilities of the worker, the worker may not be able to return to work. The occupational therapist uses skills in task adaptation to adapt or modify job tasks to allow the worker to perform the job independently. Job adaptation to increase a worker's independence or reduce exposure to ergonomic risks may involve use of adaptive equipment and work-simplification principles. A significant amount of adaptive (ergonomic) equipment is available, for example, pliers with an angled handle, which allow the user to maintain a neutral wrist position. Guidelines for ergonomic tools and handles are included in Chapter 5 of this manual.

Work-simplification principles apply to all disabilities and all aspects of occupational performance including CTDs and work. Examples of work-simplification principles that can be easily applied to the work site include the following (Trombly, 1989):

- Limit the amount of work by eliminating nonessential job tasks. This will result in energy conservation and decreased exposure to ergonomic risk factors.

- Use correct body mechanics to conserve energy and prevent injury.

- Use correct equipment. Energy is conserved, force requirements are reduced, and awkward postures are reduced if the tool fits the task.

Additional methods and strategies for adapting tasks to reduce exposure to CTD risks are included in Chapter 5, the ergonomic recommendation section of this manual.

The occupational therapist's contributions to the ergonomic team include medical knowledge, work-site experience, and communication with key professionals (e.g., physicians and insurance representatives) (Framoze, 1994). The role of the occupational therapist in this setting is as an evaluator and practitioner working to prevent work-related injuries (Jacobs, 1993). As an evaluator, the occupational therapist reviews a plant's operations to identify ergonomic risks and make ergonomic recommendations to eliminate or reduce the risks. Evaluation methods used may include records review, observation of and interview with the workers to identify ergonomic risks. As a practitioner the occupational therapist works one-to-one with workers coaching them in safe work habits.

The occupational therapist functions as a patient advocate and assists workers with developing productivity oriented attitudes and behaviors (e.g., being on time) (Mayer & Gatchel, 1988). Following an injury that results in a significant amount of time away from work, injured workers often lose their worker role identity and identify more with the patient role. They no longer feel productive. Beginning in a work-hardening program, the occupational therapist assists them with developing productivity oriented attitudes and behaviors through the use of purposeful activities (including job simulation). As the injured workers' physical capacities improve, they are able to do more and begin to feel more productive. On return to work, the occupational therapist coaches workers in safe work habits and assists them with making the final transition from the patient role to the productive worker role.

The primary focus of occupational therapists in the industrial setting is listed as follows (Mayer & Gatchel, 1988):

1. Return the patient to high functional capacity levels through work hardening and job adaptation.

2. Reduce the risk of future injuries through education sessions and job coaching.

3. Reduce pain by instructing worker in symptom management techniques.

Two ergonomic areas in which occupational therapists are uniquely qualified to address are as follows:

■ An ability to design work for an individual with special needs
■ A focus on worker safety

As a result of injury, a worker may have decreased physical capacities (special needs). Decreased physical capacities may restrict the worker from performing job duties. The occupational therapist makes recommendations for adapting and redesigning the job tasks and work station to allow the worker to perform job duties independently. Occupational therapists work to bridge the gap between the worker's capabilities and the job demands (Rice & Jacobs, 1993).

Additional Training Requirements

As discussed, occupational therapists have a background that uniquely prepares them for offering ergonomic-related services. However, this theoretical background and general training alone are not enough to prepare the occupational therapist sufficiently to provide ergonomic services. Occupational therapists need to increase their knowledge base in industrial organization and workplace politics. For example, a factory setting is much different from a hospital or clinic setting. The therapist must be familiar with the role of unions, local worker's compensation rules and regulations, marketing techniques, and appropriate employer contacts. The therapist may identify an appropriate job for a worker given his or her physical capabilities and diagnostic history. Because of the worker's low seniority, he or she will not be placed in that job. At this particular work site, the union will not allow lower seniority workers to bump higher seniority workers off jobs. It is also important to know who the appropriate contact person is at a particular work site. Generally, for worker-specific services the appropriate contact person is the supervisor or manager. For employer/company-based services the contact person is the person in charge of health and safety.

This manual is not intended to provide detailed information in industrial organization, workplace politics, and marketing industrial services. Therapists interested in providing ergonomic services are encouraged to increase their knowledge base in these areas. Suggestions for increasing knowledge base include attending related conferences, joining local organizations allowing for networking with others offering similar services, and reading related books and journals. An internship at a workplace (e.g., factory) will increase the therapist's knowledge of the workings of industrial workplaces. This experience can also increase an employer's knowledge of the field of occupational therapy and its role in ergonomics.

Occupational therapists provide many ergonomic services, including work-site risk evaluations with CTD prevention recommendations and educational sessions. This manual reviews various occupational therapy ergonomic services and offers guidelines and strategies for providing these services. Appendix A contains a list of related resources including conferences, books, journals, Internet web sites, and associations.

Guidelines for Occupational Therapy in Ergonomics

No specific guidelines have been developed for occupational therapists providing ergonomic services to business and industry. The guidelines for occupational therapists working in school systems can be used as a basis for deriving the structure of ergonomic occupational therapy guidelines. School-based occupational therapists and industrial/ business based occupational therapists are similar in many ways, including the following:

- Both are members of an interdisciplinary team.
- Both may provide services at a variety of different locations (work-sites and classrooms).
- Both provide direct services, consultative services, and monitoring services.
- Both work to achieve optimal functioning level (work skills and school skills) of their clients.
- School skills often prepare students for work and can be considered a type of work for young persons.

Dunn (1988) has described practice in the schools as consisting of three components— direct service, monitoring, and consultation. *Direct service* is when the occupational therapist provides treatment to a student/worker. An example of this type of service in ergonomics is an occupational therapist's provision of job coaching a client in proper upper extremity positioning while performing job tasks. The distinguishing characteristic of this service is that the need can only be met by direct interaction between the student/worker and the occupational therapist. The intervention requires occupational therapist's treatment techniques and ongoing clinical judgment (Dunn, 1988).

Monitoring involves teaching/supervising others in the immediate environment to carry out the treatment with the student/worker. Others in the work environment who might carry out the treatment procedures include plant nurses, safety personnel, and line supervisors. Despite the fact that the plan is being carried out by another person, the occupational therapist continues to be responsible for the outcomes. The advantage of this model is that an identified need can be best served by routine and consistent procedures. Regular contact by the occupational therapist is needed for ongoing guidance and practice. Prior to providing a monitoring service, the occupational therapist should ensure the safety of the program participants by verifying that the person conducting the program can conduct it independently, can identify program restrictions and failures, and can determine when to stop the program and contact the occupational therapist (Dunn, 1988). An example of this type of service in ergonomics is development of job rotation schedules. The occupational therapist identifies a rotation schedule that allows adequate muscle recovery time. The occupational therapist identifies jobs with different physical demands and rotates the workers through them to reduce the duration of exposure to CTD risks. Once the occupational therapist identifies the rotation schedule, it is overseen by the line supervisor who is instructed in the need for the rotation schedule, how to administer it, and what to watch for that would indicate that it is not working. The supervisor is also instructed to contact the occupational therapist when there are changes in the job demands (e.g., size of part).

Through *consultation* (Dunn, 1988), occupational therapists use specialized skills to facilitate the workings of the educational system/industrial setting. Occupational therapist consultants address problems by enabling others to work more effectively. "Consultation provides a mechanism through which students have opportunities to practice skills and generalize what they have learned to different situations" (Dunn, 1988, pp. 11–12). The key factor in consulting is the identification of a need that can be most effectively met through a change in the environment.

Dennis Isernhagen (1998) describes the following primary roles of consulting therapists in ergonomics:

- Identify client goals (e.g., decrease costs, increase production).
- Identify issues and offer cost-effective solutions.
- Develop a process not a program (ongoing).

Congruent with Dunn's explanation of consultation (Dunn, 1988) in the schools, consultation in the work environment can be directed toward the worker, the employer, and the business (system). Worker consultation (case consultation) addresses a particular worker's needs and focuses on developing a safe and effective work environment. An example of a consultation service oriented toward a particular worker is job coaching. During a job coach, the occupational therapist coaches a particular worker in safe work habits. Employer consultation (colleague consultation) assists professionals (managers) to improve their skills and knowledge. An example of a consultation service oriented toward employers is employer CTD education sessions. These sessions focus on improving a particular employer's skill and knowledge related to identifying, managing, and preventing CTDs (Dunn, 1988). Business consultation (system consultation) focuses on improving the effectiveness of the business. An example of a consultation service oriented toward the business is a risk analysis of a work setting. During a risk analysis, CTD risk factors are identified and methods for eliminating and/or reducing these risk factors are recommended. Reducing CTD risks increases the overall effectiveness of the business.

CHAPTER 5

Ergonomic Services

This section is divided into general and individual ergonomic services. The general ergonomic services are designed to meet the needs of a group, and the individual ergonomic services are designed to meet the needs of an individual.

ERGONOMIC MODIFIERS

When performing ergonomic services it is important to do a thorough review of all areas. Bob Bettendorf (1998) identifies three types of modifiers: task modifiers, personal modifiers, and psychological modifiers. These modifiers offer an ergonomic framework to assist with understanding cumulative trauma disorders (CTDs) (Claiborne & Williams, 1998).

Task modifiers, as described by Bettendorf (1998), include task designs and work methods, tool and equipment design, work-station adjustability, and the work environment (light, noise, and temperature). These areas are typically included when providing ergonomic services.

Personal modifiers refer to the worker's overall capabilities, limitations, fitness, gender, work history, and previous experience. General wellness issues are included in this modifier. Another personal modifier is worker prerogative. Worker prerogative includes posture, force applied, work speed, range of motion, repetition rate, and overexertion (Bettendorf, 1998).

Psychological modifiers include the worker's ability to cope, problem solve, and manage stress; self-esteem; and anxiety level.

When providing ergonomic services it is important to look at the person as a whole (Isenhagen et al., 1998). Omission of any of the modifiers may result in an incomplete assessment. Emphasis is typically placed only on the task itself.

PREPARING ERGONOMIC PROPOSALS

When preparing written ergonomic proposals for industry, Dan Butler (1998) recommends including the following:

- Related statistics (e.g., incidence rates for CTDs)
- Written contract or proposal
- Related fees

The following is an approximate fee list for ergonomic services. These fees may vary from state to state. Surveying fees charged by others in your area who are offering similar services is recommended.

- Risk analysis—$50.00 per work station
- Education session—$125.00 per hour or $5.00 per participant
- Job coaching and specialized work assessments—$125.00 per hour

Fees should also include mileage and report a time-cost breakdown.

SELLING OCCUPATIONAL THERAPY ERGONOMIC SERVICES TO INDUSTRY

Marketing occupational therapy services is not a major emphasis in most occupational therapy programs. Extensive marketing resources are available from other professions to assist the occupational therapist in increasing marketing knowledge and skills. Industry is often not familiar with the field of occupational therapy and its role in ergonomics. Occupational therapists offering these services must educate industry in the benefits of working with occupational therapists to reduce the incidence of CTDs.

Random cold calls to industry can be very frustrating. Targeting the companies with which the occupational therapist is already working (e.g., employer of a current acute patient with a CTD diagnosis) is often beneficial. The occupational therapist can call the employer regarding the status of the current patient and use that opportunity to introduce the other ergonomic services available. One precaution is to be sure that the patient has signed a release of information for his or her employer prior to discussing the case.

Jack Harms (1996) recommends targeting medium-size companies. He feels the people in a position of influence are more accessible. Medium-size companies are interested in decreasing costs and conserving cash flow. It is also less likely that these companies have been approached by competitors.

OCCUPATIONAL THERAPY ERGONOMIC GUIDELINES

Currently, no standards of practice exist for occupational therapists working in ergonomics. These occupational therapy ergonomic guidelines were therefore developed by the authors of this book. In general, ergonomic services consist of four components—referral, assessment, treatment or intervention program planning, and reassessment. For each of the occupational therapy ergonomic services defined in this manual (risk analysis, education sessions, specialized work assessment, job coaching, and individual worker education sessions), guidelines for each of these components are described.

GENERAL ERGONOMIC SERVICES

General ergonomic services are offered by the occupational therapist to meet the needs of the entire business. It is a general group approach, rather than an individualized approach. The general ergonomic services described in this manual include risk analysis and ergonomic education sessions. The occupational therapist providing these services functions as a consultant.

Risk Analysis

The occupational therapist, as a consultant, performs office or industrial risk analysis. During a risk analysis, the occupational therapist identifies high risk positions through review of available records. The occupational therapist then analyzes these positions for CTD risk factors through observation of workers performing various jobs and through interviews with workers and supervisors regarding job stresses. Last, the occupational therapist makes recommendations to eliminate and reduce CTD risk factors. Typically, a risk analysis is performed annually (Weber & Karen, 1998).

Referral

Risk analysis referrals are typically generated out of direct ergonomic services (e.g., job coaching and specialized work assessments). For example, during job coaching a therapist can mention to the employer the benefits of a total plant risk analysis. Using a positive job-coaching experience an occupational therapist can educate the employer in the benefits of a total plant risk analysis. The employer may then request a total plant risk analysis.

Assessment

A risk analysis assessment consists of a records review to identify high-risk positions, job analysis to identify the physical demands of the position, and risk identification.

Records Review

If available, review of OSHA Form 200 (Log and Summary of Occupational Injuries and Illness), plant medical records, worker compensation records, and payroll records would be helpful in identifying evidence of injuries or disorders associated with CTDs (Putz-Anderson, 1988). These records can be evaluated to identify the number of CTD cases and the department or job title of the injured worker. Putz-Anderson (1988) offers the following suggestions to assist with identifying CTDs through review of records.

- Most employers are required by OSHA to complete *OSHA Form 200 logs* (Log and Summary of Occupational Injuries and Illnesses). Employers are required to document all on-the-job illnesses and injuries. The OSHA Form 200 log is the standard form for keeping work-related injury and illness records. Item 7f is the repeated trauma category. This category includes disorders associated with repeated motion, vibration, pressure, and hearing loss. By scanning this column, cases of CTDs can be identified along with the corresponding department (column E), job title (column D), and date of injury (column B). Plant departments with high numbers of CTDs can be identified. The date of injury may provide insight into the effects of procedure or equipment changes.

- Larger plants may have their own medical departments. Visits to this department are often recorded in the employees' *medical file*. Medical file entries typically include the same information as the OSHA Form 200, a description of the medical treatment given and work restrictions. All medical records should be regarded as confidential. Through review of these records, cases of CTDs may be identified. It may be difficult to review the significant number of files at a large plant unless the records are recorded on a computer file that is accessible through data base software. Random sampling techniques may also be used to identify CTD cases.

- The associated costs of CTDs (medical expenses and disability payments) as well as the departments and job titles where the costs of CTDs are high can be identified through review of *worker's compensation insurance records*. The costs documented on these records do not include medical treatments provided directly by the employer. The section on injury description can be checked to identify cases of CTDs.

- *Payroll records* can be reviewed to identify departments and job titles with high absenteeism and turnover rates. Workers commonly leave jobs that are physically stressful by quitting or transferring to another department.

The usefulness of the record review in identifying the incident rates of CTDs is dependent on how well the information is recorded by the employer. The clearer and more thorough the records are, the more accurate the information obtained (Putz-Anderson, 1988).

These records may not be available for review by the occupational therapist since many are considered confidential and the occupational therapist is working as a consultant and not as an employee of the company. If the occupational therapist is not able or allowed to review the records, the occupational therapist should ask the employer to review the OSHA Form 200 logs to identify the departments and job titles with a high incidence of CTDs. The occupational therapist can then use time effectively and focus on the identified departments and jobs when analyzing CTD risks and making ergonomic recommendations.

Job Analysis to Identify CTD Risks

A job analysis is defined as an organized procedure for describing the tasks and conditions of a job (Jacobs, 1989). A job is described as a set of tasks, each task is defined in a series of steps or elements, and the elements are described as movements required to perform the job (Putz-Anderson, 1988). A job analysis is a two-stage process consisting of task analysis and risk identification.

Task Analysis

Task analysis involves breaking down a job into its component parts. The steps required to perform the jobs are identified through observation and interviews with the worker and supervisor. The movements involved or acts performed (e.g., grasping, bending, turning, cutting flash, and flipping part) are documented. Several different people should be observed performing the same job to identify any differences in technique, style, and rate, as job risks can be influenced by worker style and technique. The job analysis should evaluate the work station (furniture and machinery in the work space), hand tools (power and manual tools), equipment used (personal protective equipment and jigs), parts and materials involved, work methods (postures and movements), and environmental conditions (noise level, lighting, and temperature). Weights, distances, heights, force required, and rate/production for a particular job should be documented (Kasdan, 1991). Whether or not the worker has control over the technique, style, and rate should be evaluated (e.g., how the worker holds the part).

If possible, the job should be videotaped recording several complete cycles of the operation for future reference and reevaluation. The videotape should include the name and location of the facility, name of the evaluator, and the date and time of day. The whole body of the worker as well as a close-up of the worker's upper extremities should be videotaped. Tape from different angles, if possible, to focus on particular upper extremity motions (Kasdan, 1991). Prior to videotaping, it may be necessary to have the workers who are to be taped sign a written consent to be photographed.

When going to the work site, it is important to wear clothing that is appropriate for that setting. An office setting demands significantly different attire from a factory. Plant and factory floors are often oily and dirty; therefore, rubber-soled shoes are recommended. Prior to going to the work site, it is beneficial to ask the contact person if there are any clothing and safety equipment requirements at the job site (e. g., hard hats, safety glasses, steel-toed shoes, ear plugs). Table 5–1 contains a list of suggested equipment to bring to the job site when evaluating job demands.

Table 5–1. A list of equipment that may be needed when performing an on-site job analysis.

Ear plugs	Video camera and film
Tape measure	Dictaphone and tapes
Distance-measuring device	Scale
Camera and film	Force gauge

Risk Identification

Following the job analysis, each task is analyzed to identify potential CTD risk factors. "A risk factor is defined as an attribute or exposure that increases the probability of the disease or disorder" (Putz-Anderson, 1988, pp. 49–50). Force, repetition, and posture are considered the primary risk factors (Kasdan, 1991). The University of Michigan Center for Occupational Health and Safety Engineering has developed guidelines for rating work-related risk factors (Ulin, 1997). The CTD risk factors are listed and defined below.

■ *Repetitive tasks* with insufficient muscle recovery time may result in CTDs (Grandjean, 1988). Repetitive tasks require rapid and frequent muscle contractions. Frequent muscle contractions can cause a decrease in muscle tension, resulting in increased muscle effort needed to perform the task (Putz-Anderson, 1988). When evaluating repetitiveness, the number of cycles occurring during a shift are counted. Repetition = cycles/hour. The shorter the cycle time, the more repetitive the job is. Cycle times shorter than 30 seconds (1000 or more cycles per 8-hour shift) are considered to be highly repetitive. Fundamental cycles can also be assessed to determine the repetitiveness of a job. Fundamental cycles are repeated sets of motions within a cycle. Jobs are considered highly repetitive when 50% of the cycle time is spent performing the same fundamental cycle (Kasdan, 1991). An example of a repetitive task is engine assembly line work. The assembly line worker is required to place a small (6 ounce) circular part on an engine. The worker uses one hand to place the part on the engine while the other hand retrieves the parts from a bin to the worker's right. Production is 2000 repetitions per hour with a cycle time of 33 seconds. The job would be considered highly repetitive and may result in a CTD.

■ *Awkward postures* are defined as constrained body positions. End-range (i.e., extreme) joint positions are considered awkward postures. An example of an end-range posture is full wrist flexion (80°). These postures cause biomechanical joint and soft tissue stress. Postures are considered poor when they overload the muscles and tendons, load joints asymmetrically, or involve a static load on the musculature. Muscle strength decreases proportionally as the joint deviates from neutral (Putz-Anderson, 1988). Table 5–2 shows the proportional percentage of grip strength as the wrist deviates from neutral.
    Examples of awkward postures at various joints are as follows:

1. Hand—pinching with thumb and index fingertip pulps (three jaw and tip-to-tip pinch)
2. Wrist—extreme flexion, extension, ulnar deviation, and radial deviation

Table 5–2. The proportional decrease in grip strength as the wrist deviates from neutral (Putz-Anderson, 1998).

Wrist Position	Percent of Grip Strength
Neutral	100
Radial deviation	80
Ulnar deviation	75
Extension	75
Flexion	45

Table 5–3. Common CTDs and postures to avoid (Cannon, 1991).

Cumulative Trauma Disorder	Posture to Avoid
Carpal tunnel syndrome	Wrist flexion, extension, and deviation, sustained pinch and grip
Cubital tunnel syndrome	Pressure on elbows, repetitive elbow flexion and extension, prolonged elbow flexion
Radial tunnel syndrome	Forceful/repetitive wrist extension, forceful or repetitive supination, palm-down lifts
Thoracic outlet syndrome	Sustained above-shoulder-level activity
De Quervain's disease	Combination of thumb flexion, wrist ulnar deviation, and wrist flexion; forceful pinching
Flexor carpi ulnaris tendinitis	Repetitive wrist ulnar deviation and flexion
Lateral epicondylitis (tennis elbow)	Palm-down lifts, forcible elbow extension, supination, and wrist extension; forceful wrist and elbow extension with forearms pronated
Trigger finger/trigger thumb	Repetitive grasping, power grip

3. Elbow—extreme flexion, extension, pronation, and supination

4. Shoulder—reaching above shoulder level and reaching down and behind the torso (hyperextension)

5. Neck and back—forward head posture and extreme trunk flexion

Awkward postures are evaluated by observation of a worker performing job tasks and/or reviewing a videotape of the job. Table 5–3 lists common CTDs and postures to avoid. It is more accurate to record the number of awkward postures from a videotape (Kasdan, 1991).

■ A *static contraction* is the prolonged state of contraction of a muscle. During a static contraction, a metabolic imbalance is produced within the muscle. Internal pressure of the muscle tissues compresses blood vessels and decreases blood flow (Isernhagen, S. J., 1998). The muscle's supply of oxygen and nutrients are depleted and waste products are not excreted. Muscle pain and fatigue occur during static contractions (Grandjean, 1988). Putz-Anderson (1988) defines work conditions that require excessive static hand-arm effort as slight effort lasting 10 seconds or longer, moderate effort lasting 1 minute or longer, and high effort lasting 4 minutes or longer. Greater hold time requires greater rest time (Isernhagen, S. J., 1998). An example of a task requiring static muscle contraction is carrying a box at waist level in both hands 50 feet. The upper extremity muscles holding the box while the box is being carried across the room are in static contraction.

■ *Force* required to perform job tasks is a contributing factor to CTDs. Heavy loads require greater muscle effort and cause a decrease in muscle circulation. Muscles exerting excessive force fatigue more rapidly and may require greater muscle recovery time than work time. Lack of sufficient muscle recovery time can result in soft tissue injuries (Putz-Anderson, 1988). Force can be evaluated through observation of the grip posture, documentation of the object's weight, duration of the action, and location of the load. More sophisticated methods are available for force analysis (e.g., electromyography to measure muscle activity and thin pressure sensitive force devices that are attached to gloves). These devices require some expertise to use and the equipment may not be practical when evaluating a large number of jobs (Kasdan, 1991). Acceptable force limits vary for different body parts, and they are influenced by age, sex, body build, and general health (Putz-Anderson, 1988). An example of a job that requires excessive force is a material-handling position that requires the worker to lift large and bulky objects weighing up to 100 pounds off a shelf above shoulder level and place them on the floor.

■ *Gloves* that are poorly fitting result in increased hand force requirements and, therefore, increased stress on the worker. Gloves may also decrease the coefficient of friction between the hand and the objects held and/or desensitize the hand receptors, causing the worker to grip harder (greater muscle effort) than needed to perform the job task (Kasdan, 1991). However, some gloves may increase the coefficient of friction and make it easier to grip smooth objects (e.g., the use of rubber gloves to open a jar) (Pheasant, 1991). The effects of gloves can be evaluated through observation.

■ *Contact pressure/mechanical stress* can affect the palm, sides and backs of fingers, forearm, elbow, and axillary region. Tendons and nerves can be injured from contact pressure/mechanical stress. Mechanical stress is the result of contact with hard, sharp edges, including tool handles, work surfaces, and parts. Sources of mechanical stress can be identified through observation (Kasdan, 1991). Examples of contact pressure/mechanical stress include pressure at the base of the palm when depressing palm buttons, pressure on the volar surface of the forearm when leaning against a sharp-edged workbench, and scissors rubbing the sides of fingers compressing the digit digital nerves.

■ *Vibration* causes blood vessels to constrict and may eventually damage the nerves of the fingers. Constricted blood vessels result in muscle oxygen and nerve deprivation (Putz-Anderson, 1988). Vibration may also result in soft tissue microtrauma and scarring. If possible, the frequency and the power of vibration should be evaluated (Kasdan, 1991). Power tools with vibration frequencies between 40 and 300 Hz can have ill effects on the blood vessels and nerves of the hands (Grandjean, 1988). Vibration may also desensitize the hand receptors and cause the worker to grip harder. An example of a vibration risk is use of a pneumatic drill with excessive vibration.

■ *Cold temperatures* can result in soft tissue stiffness, constricted blood vessels (decreased circulation), and decreased sensation (Kasdan, 1991). This reduced sensitivity may result in the worker exerting five times more force than necessary to perform the job task (Armstrong, 1994). A thermometer can be used to evaluate temperature. The temperature of the worker's environment as well as objects held (e.g., tools and parts) should be assessed. Exposure of the hand to work objects or air temperature below 20° Celsius (68° Fahrenheit) is considered a CTD risk (Armstrong, 1994). Meat cutters who work in refrigerated environments may be at risk of developing CTDs.

Many risk factors are associated with various disorders. Table 5–4 identifies the risk factors and gives examples of disorders commonly associated with them.

Intervention Planning

Following identification of CTD risk factors, the occupational therapy consultant makes recommendations for eliminating or reducing these risks. The recommendations are typically not carried out by the occupational therapist. They are given to the employer who decides whether or not to follow through with the recommendations.

Ergonomic Recommendations

These recommendations should be cost effective, feasible, and practical. Frequently, minor and inexpensive changes can result in a significant decrease in CTD risks. It is often difficult to get the support needed to implement expensive and time-consuming changes. However, some expensive ergonomic recommendations are cost effective in the long run. The cost of the recommended change can be compared with the cost of injury (Kasdan, 1991).

The most obvious risk factors should be addressed first. Since the primary risk factors are force, repetition, and posture, these factors should be reduced or eliminated first. Efforts should be made to eliminate situations that lead to awkward postures, reduce the amount of force needed, and reduce the number of repetitions needed to complete the task (Kasdan, 1991). Appendix B includes an example of a portion of a risk analysis report

Table 5–4. Risk factors and examples of disorders commonly associated with them (Putz-Anderson, 1988).

Risk Factor	Disorder
Repetition	Carpal tunnel syndrome and tenosynovitis
Awkward posture	Extreme wrist flexion/extension—carpal tunnel syndrome Wrist ulnar and radial deviation—De-Quervain's disease Above-shoulder-level reaching—thoracic outlet syndrome
Static contraction	Degenerative tendinitis and tenosynovitis
Force	Forceful gripping—trigger finger
Vibration	Occupational Raynaud's

that identifies risks and makes ergonomic recommendations for reducing and/or eliminating these identified risks.

Engineering solutions and administrative solutions can be used to reduce CTD risk factors.

Engineering Solutions

Engineering solutions include redesigning the environment, work station, tools and equipment, materials and parts, and work methods. These solutions are related to the workplace layout. The best way to remove CTD risk factors is to design the work station to fit human measurements. Anthropometrics is an area of ergonomics that studies body measurements (Pheasant, 1991). Anthropometric data (human body size data) can be used to design work stations that accommodate 90% of the population. These data are available in various ergonomic books and typically are in chart form. Designing for the average is not recommended because this work station will not accommodate larger and smaller people. It is better to design for the extremes, accommodating larger and smaller people. Adjustable work stations can accommodate a large variety of people (Kasdan, 1991).

WORK STATIONS. The work station can be redesigned to reduce exposure to force and posture risks. Forceful exertions can be decreased by reducing the weight of tools and objects and by ensuring optimal mechanical advantage. The postural risk of excessive upper extremity reaching is reduced by relocating needed items to within safe reaching distances (Kasdan, 1991). Suggestions for reducing CTD risks by redesigning the work station are as follows (Putz-Anderson, 1988):

- Design work stations that can adjust to accommodate the majority of the workers.
- To avoid prolonged static muscle loading, design a work station that allows the worker to change positions frequently (e.g., sit and stand option).
- Reduce the amount of excessive upper extremity reaching by placing tools, equipment, and materials between shoulder and waist level.
- The work surface for heavy work should be at a lower level than for precise work.
- Be sure the chair is well designed and fits the worker and the job. An adjustable chair (seat height, back rest, and foot rest) is recommended.

TOOLS AND HANDLES. A well-designed tool increases productivity and reduces CTD risks. Many workers customize their own tools to improve the effectiveness and comfort of the tool. Observations of the ways workers have adapted their tools can provide insight into ways to redesign tools to reduce risk and increase effectiveness. Putz-Anderson (1988) recommends the following be avoided when designing tools and handles: high contact forces (e.g., sharp edges), static muscle loading, end-range joint postures, repetitive finger motion, and tool vibration. The following is a list of recommended guidelines for tool selection and design (Putz-Anderson, 1988):

- The worker should be provided with handles to grip rather than grasping the tool's surface. The tool handles should reduce exposure to vibration, cool air currents, and skin burns. The handle should improve tool control while increasing the mechanical advantage.

- The tool should require minimal muscular effort to use. Tool suspension systems are beneficial. They allow the worker to let go of the tool between work cycles and often support the weight of the tool. The tool should be balanced with its center of gravity located close to the tool's body to reduce fatigue.

- To reduce human force and repetition requirements, tools should be powered with motors rather than muscles.

- Choose tools with handles that allow for neutral (straight) wrist positioning. Many tools have been designed with bent handles that are most effective when all the work is done in one plane. The tool may allow for a straight wrist position when working in one plane and require end-range wrist positioning when working in another plane.

- Trigger strips (using index and middle fingers) are preferred over trigger buttons because they reduce finger muscle fatigue.

- The weight of most frequently used tools should be kept low. Tools that weigh more than 2 pounds should be supported by a counterbalancing harness. An exception to this rule is that some power tools are easier to operate if they are heavier because the operator does not have to exert as much force to provide even pressure on the surface (e.g., buffers and grinders).

- Develop special purpose tools for the task rather than having the operator adapt to a standard tool.

- Tools should be designed for use in either hand.

- When significant human force is required, the handle should be designed for a power grip. A power grip is more efficient and less fatiguing. Precision (pinch) grips should be avoided because they are inefficient and fatiguing.

- Tool handles should be the proper size for the worker. Cylindrical or oval handles are recommended. Textured rubber handles and T-shaped handles allow for greater torque with less grip force.

- The tool should be at least 4 inches long to avoid contact pressure at the base of the palm.

- Form-fitted handles often do not fit the majority of hand sizes and often cause the fingers to stretch apart. Grip ability is decreased because it is difficult to flex the fingers when they are spread apart (i.e., abduction).

- Tool surfaces should be slip resistant.

WORK METHODS. Putz-Anderson (1988) identified guidelines for redesigning work methods to reduce and eliminate CTD risk factors. His guidelines include the use of jigs and fixtures to hold parts rather than the worker gripping and holding the part, job enlargement (i.e., combine jobs) to reduce repetition, automation of highly repetitive jobs to allow some worker control over the work pace, allowing new workers to start at a slow pace to become conditioned to work tasks, job task rotation, and encouraging frequent rest breaks (muscle recovery time).

Administrative Solutions

Administrative solutions include training and educating, the creation of exercise and conditioning programs for workers, job rotation, and job enlargement. Occupational therapists are instrumental in recommending and implementing administrative solutions. Job rotation is defined as "systematically changing the person from one job to another" (Kasdan, 1991, p. 554). The purpose of rotation is to reduce exposure to CTD risk factors. The physical demands of the jobs that workers are rotated through must be physically different to reduce exposure to CTD risks (Putz-Anderson, 1988). Job enlargement is defined as "adding more work content to the job to reduce the frequency of a particular stress" (Kasdan, 1991, p. 554).

Repetitiveness can be reduced through rate reduction, job enlargement, and job rotation. Force and postural stresses can be reduced by decreasing the number of objects held and distributing workloads over large body parts. Through education and training, tasks can be modified to reduce and eliminate exposure to CTD risk factors (Kasdan, 1991).

Reassessment

It is recommended that a total plant or office risk analysis be completed yearly. During the annual risk analysis, the effects of previously recommended interventions can be analyzed as well as identifying new ergonomic risks. A risk analysis on a particular job or department may be done more frequently if there has been a significant increase in the number of injuries on that position, or if new machinery or equipment has been installed.

Education Sessions

Ergonomic education sessions focus on improving the employer's and worker's knowledge and skill level as related to CTD identification, prevention, and management. The goal of these education sessions is to assist industry with developing in-house knowledge to enable problem identification and resolution (Kasdan, 1991). Education sessions are tailored to meet the specific needs of the different levels of the organization (i.e., managers, engineering and design personnel, supervisors, and workers).

The occupational therapist's philosophical and theoretical foundation uniquely prepares them for providing ergonomic education sessions. The theoretical role of the occupational therapist is to facilitate learning of skills and functions needed for adaptation and production and to promote and maintain health (Dutton, 1993). When providing businesses with ergonomic education sessions, the occupational therapist is teaching the participants the skills and functions needed to adapt their environment to reduce the risk of injury. The occupational therapist is promoting health and injury prevention (wellness).

Referral

Referral for an ergonomic education and training session is typically generated out of direct ergonomic services or may be a risk analysis recommendation. Other referral sources may include attorneys, insurance companies, physicians, and clinical therapists. The occupational therapist can educate the employer about the benefits of education sessions while providing other ergonomic services. Occasionally employers independently request the education service. The occupational therapist functions as a consultant when providing ergonomic education and training.

Assessment

The ergonomic education assessment simply consists of identifying the educational needs of the employees. This is done through interview with the employer contact person. Questions the occupational therapist may want to ask the contact person include:

- What are the different organizational levels of the company?
- What is the educational background of the employees for the different organizational levels?
- Will the training session be voluntary or mandatory for the employees?
- Approximately how many employees will participate in the training session?

Intervention

Management and workers should be trained in the skills needed to recognize job hazards and methods for reducing these identified hazards. All levels of the organization (management, engineering, supervisors, and workers) should be included in the ergonomic education program. Since there is a significant amount of background diversity at the various levels of the organization (i.e., experience, abilities, educational background, focus, and function), separate sessions designed to meet the needs of the specific level should be offered. All educational programs should include discussion of anatomy, biomechanics, CTD risk factors, and ergonomic principles tailored to meet the needs of the various groups (Kasdan, 1991).

Lecturing is the training method frequently used. An advantage of lectures is that they are practical. A large amount of information can be given to a large number of people in a short amount of time. The lecture content can be tailored to meet the group's specific needs. The lectures can be enhanced with visual aides (e.g., slides and still photos) and props (e.g., anatomical models, gloves, and ergonomic equipment). Slides and videotape presentations can be used to demonstrate the difference between safe and unsafe work habits. Slides and videos of the participants' actual jobs can lead to group discussion for risk identification and resolution. Information should be presented in a way that can be easily transferred to the workplace.

Table 5–5 provides an overview of Kasdan's (1991) recommended content for the educational programs for the various groups. A brief description of the content and focus of lectures at the various levels is as follows:

- The ergonomic lecture aimed at *managers* should include a broad range of ergonomic issues. The lecture topics should include CTD incidence, prevalence, and associated employer costs; plant CTD surveillance approaches; injury medical management; return-to-work options following an injury; recommendation feasibility; and labor and union issues. Administrative controls should be discussed (Kasdan, 1991). The primary emphasis of management education programs should be to increase knowledge of and commitment to ergonomics, resulting in adequate resource support (Armstrong, 1994).

- The ergonomic lectures for *engineering and design personnel* should introduce the human element to their existing technical and scientific backgrounds. Engineers and design personnel can be instructed in ergonomic principles that will allow them to design new jobs and redesign existing positions to reduce and eliminate CTD risk factors. Topics covered may include posture as it relates to the height of the work surface, handle design for optimal strength, assistive devices to reduce force requirements and awkward postures, and the effects of vibration (Kasdan, 1991). Engineers can be taught how to recognize stressful work designs and can be helpful with designing interventions (Armstrong, 1994).

- *Supervisors* should be taught how to recognize and avoid CTD risks. Job-specific examples can be used to teach the skills needed for the identification of CTD risk

Table 5–5. Educational program content for various groups.

Group	Educational Program Content
Managers	Prevalence, incidence, and employer costs of CTDs Injury surveillance approaches Existing injury medical management approaches Worker reentry following an injury Productivity implications Labor union issues Administrative controls
Engineering and design personnel	Introduce the human element to their existing scientific and technical knowledge base Exertional forces related to body parts Performance capabilities related to pacing Handle designs for optimal strength Physiological effects of vibration Safe reaching and lifting parameters Gloves Assistive devices
Supervisors	Recognition and avoidance of risks Effective and safe worker training
Workers	Self-protection and personal safety responsibility Risk recognition and avoidance

factors. Group problem solving should be encouraged to give participants the opportunity to practice identifying hazards and implementing safe work practices. Examples of safe work practices that supervisors can implement include proper tool use, the proper structure for job rotation, placement of controls parts and materials, and training of workers in work safety (Kasdan, 1991). Supervisors that are taught how to recognize and report work hazards will be more cooperative with intervention measures (Armstrong, 1991).

■ *Worker* education sessions should emphasize the importance of taking responsibility for one's own safety. The workers should be aware of their responsibility for self-protection. The responsibility for worker safety is equally shared between the employer and employee. For example, the employer can encourage safe work methods, but the employee has to follow through with these methods. Workers who are involved in the ergonomic process are more likely to accept the recommended changes. The workers should also be instructed in risk identification (hazardous motions and activities) and in avoidance of risky work habits. Group discussion to identify job-specific risks is beneficial. The goal of worker education sessions is not only to give the workers the knowledge but also to give them the skills needed to identify and avoid risks. Workers may need to be taught new methods for completing familiar tasks. They must be coached to overcome undesirable habits and to acquire new habits. The worker will need practice and feedback to learn and become comfortable with new work habits (Kasdan, 1991).

Policies for return-to-work programs, modified jobs, and reporting procedures for early diagnosis should be clearly defined and augment the education programs. A plan for early intervention should exist. Appendix C contains sample ergonomic educational and training handouts.

Reassessment

The ergonomic education sessions should be offered yearly to existing employees and quarterly for new employees. The purpose of yearly sessions is to review the ergonomic material to refresh the employees memories. This will continue to encourage them to avoid and report risks. It will also demonstrate management's ongoing commitment to safety.

INDIVIDUAL ERGONOMIC SERVICES

Individual ergonomic services are offered by the occupational therapist for a particular worker. These direct occupational therapist work-site services include specialized work assessments/worker-specific job analysis, job coaching, and individual worker education sessions. The following description of these services is based on the first author's experience providing these services at Michigan Hand Rehabilitation Center in Dearborn, Michigan.

Specialized Work Assessment

A specialized work assessment is a worker-specific job analysis. It is similar to a risk analysis; however, it is focused on one worker's position only. The purpose of a specialized work assessment is to identify the physical demands of the worker's job, identify any risks and hazards (particularly as they relate to the worker's diagnosis), make ergonomic recommendations to reduce and eliminate the risk factors identified, make ergonomic equipment recommendations, and draw conclusions regarding whether or not this would be a feasible job for the worker based on the diagnosis and his or her physical capabilities. A specialized work assessment typically lasts 1 to 2 hours depending on the number of job tasks. This time does not include travel time and report time.

Specialized work assessments are tailored to assess the physical requirements of a specific worker's position as it relates to the worker's physical capabilities and diagnostic history. Risks are identified as they relate to the worker's diagnosis and recommendations are made for resolving the risks. If it is determined the position is not feasible for return to work, an attempt is made to identify alternative positions that are within the worker's physical capabilities and restrictions. Because each specialized work assessment is different, no standardized form is available for documenting this service. Please refer to Appendix D for a sample specialized work assessment report and a sample report template.

Referral

The referral for this service is typically generated by the physician, treating therapist, attorney, case manager, insurance representative, and/or rehabilitation nurse. A physician's prescription is not needed for this service because it is an evaluation not a treatment. A specialized work assessment is often recommended for a worker with a history of CTDs, who is typically not working because of an injury. Following acute medical treatment, a specialized work assessment may be necessary to assist with safely returning an injured worker to work. Information gathered can be used to develop a return-to-work plan and identify any accommodations needed.

Assessment

Specific guidelines for the assessment portion of a specialized work assessment are as follows:

1. The occupational therapist should phone the worker prior to the specialized work assessment to get the worker's impression of job demands and physical stresses. The worker's description can be compared with the employer's description. The therapist should phone the employer contact to set up time, get directions, and identify dress and safety equipment requirements

2. The occupational therapist meets with the manager and/or supervisor to discuss return-to-work options. It is also beneficial to have the manager describe the worker's position, which gives the occupational therapist the opportunity to document unfamiliar terms (e.g., part names and tools used). Since many job sites are very noisy it may be beneficial to ask the manager the above questions in an office or quiet space. Questions the occupational therapist may want to ask the manager include the following:

   ■ Are modified or light duty positions available?

   ■ Can the worker return to work on a graded schedule?

   ■ What are the work hours and when are the scheduled breaks (e.g., lunch)?

   ■ Is overtime mandatory?

   ■ Are there production demands/quotas/incentives?

   ■ Are there labor unions?

3. The occupational therapist then goes to the work station and observes a worker performing the job tasks. As with a risk analysis, videos and still photos are helpful with recording cycles, movement patterns, and work habits. Use of a small hand-held dictaphone may be helpful with orally recording the job demands, risks, and possible recommendations. Interviewing the worker and the supervisor is also beneficial with identifying job demands and risk factors. The occupational therapist documents the job demands, including pertinent heights, weights, and measurements. If possible, it is beneficial for the occupational therapist to perform the job to get hands on experience regarding the physical stresses encountered.

4. The occupational therapist documents any risks identified during the specialized work assessment. Any job tasks that require physical demands that may be contraindicated for the worker's diagnosis should be identified. For example, a worker with a diagnosis of bilateral carpal tunnel syndrome may have a job that requires her to flex her wrist several times an hour to retrieve a part from the press. Frequent end-range wrist flexion is a known contributing factor to carpal tunnel syndrome.

Appendix D contains a specialized work assessment sample report.

Intervention Planning

Intervention planning consists of formulating worker-specific ergonomic recommendations based on the results of the assessment. The following are guidelines for specialized work assessment intervention planning:

1. The final report should include a plan for reducing and/or eliminating worker-specific risk factors that were identified during the assessment. Recommendations for adaptive and/or ergonomic equipment needed should be made. Worker education sessions and job coaching are common specialized work assessment recommendations.

2. The report should also include conclusions regarding the feasibility of the worker returning to work at the current position given the diagnosis.

3. If it is concluded that the job reviewed would not be an appropriate return-to-work position for the worker, alternative return-to-work positions with the same employer can be identified.

4. Following the work assessment, the occupational therapist should make case management calls to involved parties (i.e., physician, insurance representative, and/or rehabilitation specialist) to give a verbal report of the results of the specialized work assessment; the calls should be followed by a written report. Recommendations are discussed with the referral source and arrangements are made for additional ergonomic services (e.g., job coaching and worker education sessions).

The information obtained during the specialized work assessment has various uses. The physician uses the information to determine if there is a match between the worker's capabilities, diagnosis, and job demands. Based on the job demands, the physician determines whether or not work restrictions are necessary. The treating therapist may use the information to set up job simulations in the clinic. In the clinic, the injured worker performs simulated job tasks to improve work tolerances. The therapist can also make comparisons between the job demands and the injured worker's physical capabilities as demonstrated during therapy or during a functional capacity evaluation.

Reassessment

A specialized work assessment is typically a one-time service. However, reassessment may be necessary if workers' job demands change or if they are transferred to a different position. A different position may have different ergonomic risk factors. A reassessment may also be necessary if there is a change in workers' physical capabilities.

Job Coaching

The purpose of job coaching, in the context of treating upper extremity CTDs, is to encourage upper extremity wellness in the workplace. The worker is coached by the occupational therapist to perform tasks using safe work habits. A job-coaching session typically lasts 1 hour. This does not include report time and travel time.

Referral

The referral for job coaching is typically generated by the physician, treating therapist, employer, or rehabilitation specialist. Job coaching is often recommended for an injured worker who has been released by a physician to return to work following time off work as a result of an injury. Job coaching may also be beneficial for a worker who is experiencing beginning CTD symptoms or a worker with a history of CTDs who is being transferred to a different position.

Assessment

The recommended guidelines for a job-coaching assessment are as follows:

■ The occupational therapist observes the worker performing all job tasks. A brief description of job demands is documented. Videotapes or still photos of the worker performing job duties are recommended.

■ The occupational therapist interviews the worker and supervisor regarding job demands, physical stresses, and risks.

Appendix E contains a job coach sample report and sample report template.

Intervention

The occupational therapist observes a worker performing job tasks and provides feedback regarding proper upper extremity posturing and pacing. The occupational therapist may also make simple changes in the setup of the work station to reduce and/or eliminate upper extremity risk factors. Recommended guidelines for completing the intervention portion of job coaching are listed bellow:

1. The worker is coached to perform tasks using new and safer work habits. Particular emphasis is placed on performing tasks with midrange upper extremity positioning and pacing of activities whenever possible. The occupational therapist may demonstrate the new work habit to the worker followed by frequent verbal coaching and positive reinforcement while the worker practices these movements.

2. The worker is instructed in simple warm-up exercises and is encouraged to perform these exercises prior to beginning work and frequently throughout the workday. These exercises include simple range-of-motion exercises for the neck, upper extremities, back, and lower extremities. Particular emphasis is placed on stretching and warming up the muscles frequently used to perform job tasks.

3. The occupational therapist may make simple changes to the work-station to reduce or eliminate upper extremity risk factors. Simple work-station changes may include relocation of equipment and/or supplies to reduce upper extremity reaching and awkward postures.

4. The occupational therapist may instruct the worker in symptom management techniques, including the use of cold packs during breaks. Cold packs are placed over the painful area with a towel between the pack and skin. The cold pack is left on 15 to 20 minutes until the skin becomes numb. The stages of cold are cold → ache → burn → numb. The occupational therapist should be trained in the use of physical agent modalities prior to administering them.

5. The occupational therapist makes additional recommendations for ergonomic equipment and work-station redesign needs.

6. The worker's response to job coaching should be documented (e.g., Was the worker resistant or open to the occupational therapist's suggestions? Did the worker appear to be following through with the therapist's recommendations?).

Reassessment

Job coaching is typically a one-time service. If the worker appears to be having difficulty incorporating new and safer work habits, a second job coaching session may be necessary to reinforce new work habits. A second job coach may also be necessary if the job demands or position change. A different position will have different physical demands and movement patterns. The worker may require guidance in incorporating safe work habits at the new position.

Individual Worker Education Sessions

Referral

The referral for an individual worker education session is typically generated by the physician, worker, employer, treating therapist, or rehabilitation specialist. This education session is most effective when provided prior to job coaching. This education session is typically recommended for workers with a history of CTDs. This session is also beneficial for workers experiencing beginning CTD symptoms. It is often recommended when group education sessions are not offered or when the worker's needs can best be met by a one-to-one session.

Assessment

The worker is interviewed to identify his or her current symptoms and methods for controlling symptoms. Typical questions include the following

- Point to where it hurts.
- What makes you feel worse?
- What makes you feel better?
- Is there any pattern to your symptoms?

Workers are also asked to offer a brief description of their job demands and perceived physical stresses of their job. Commonly asked questions are listed below:

- Describe your job.
- Demonstrate the motions you use on your job.
- Do you lift/carry anything on your job? If yes, how much does it weigh?
- Do you use any tools on your job?
- What are the physical stresses of your job?
- Do you have any suggestions for reducing the physical stresses of your job?

Intervention

This service is offered either at the work site or in the clinic. A quiet room with minimal distractions is recommended. As with group worker education sessions, visual aides and props enhance the session. The material covered during this education session is very similar to the information covered in the group session. However, greater emphasis is placed on the worker's diagnosis and job tasks. Specific information covered may include the following:

- The worker is given a brief description of CTDs and the type of CTD affecting him or her. A description of other types of CTDs is *not* given. If the specific diagnosis for the worker is not known, diagnosis is not discussed during the session.

■ The worker is instructed in the importance of avoiding end-range joint positions. The worker is encouraged to perform tasks using midrange joint positions at work and at home.

■ The worker is encouraged to pace him- or herself during tasks whenever possible. Emphasis is placed on the importance of taking frequent short breaks throughout the day rather than rushing through tasks, then taking a break at the end.

■ If available, the therapist and worker view a videotape of the worker performing job tasks. Through discussion, awkward postures are identified, and the worker is encouraged to problem solve to identify safer work postures. If a videotape of the worker is not available, the worker is asked to demonstrate the physical stresses of his or her job and problem solve to identify alternative techniques.

■ Pain management techniques and principles are discussed, including the use of cold packs if the occupational therapist has had training in the use of this physical agent modality.

Reassessment

An individual worker education session is typically a one-time service. Following the initial one-to-one session, the worker can participate in yearly group education sessions, if available, to reinforce injury prevention techniques and principles. Group education sessions are much more cost effective. If the employer does not wish to provide yearly group education sessions, yearly individual follow-up sessions can be recommended.

CHAPTER 6

Cumulative Trauma Disorders and Computer Keyboard Users

INCIDENCE FOR COMPUTER USERS

There is a steady rise in the incidence of cumulative trauma disorders (CTDs) for computer keyboard users. The bureau of labor statistics survey revealed that 12% of work-related CTDs were attributed to typing or key entry (Bureau of Labor Statistics, 1994). Approximately one half of all workers (60 million Americans) use computers on a daily basis (Keller et al., 1998).

RISK FACTORS FOR COMPUTER USERS

CTD risk factors for computer users are similar to the general risk factors discussed in Chapter 5. This section reviews common CTD risks as they relate to computer users.

Keller and colleagues (1998) identify the following CTD risk factors for computer users.

- Work pace/repetition—lack of rest breaks and muscle recovery, high typing rate, and deadlines
- Awkward postures—from incompatible work surface heights, poor chair support, and worker habits
- Excessive force—key striking
- Static loading/posturing—lack of upper extremity support
- Contact pressure—sharp work surface edges, stapler, and scissor finger holes

When assessing a worker's posture at the computer, it is important to observe the head, neck, and shoulder posture in addition to end-range upper extremity posturing. Poor posture at the computer typically consists of forward head posture and forward rolled shoulders. Other postural concerns for computer users include wrist ulnar deviation, hyperflexion, and hyperextension and finger malalignments. These end range postures (repetitive and static) compromise joint mechanics and muscle length tension relationships, possibly resulting in CTDs (Keller et al., 1998).

COMMON CTD DIAGNOSIS FOR COMPUTER USERS

Many common upper extremity CTDs have been recognized among computer users. Keller and coworkers (1998) divide computer user CTDs by anatomical location. Table 6–1 lists the various diagnoses by anatomical location and awkward posture.

EVALUATION OF CTD RISKS FOR COMPUTER USERS

Workers should be evaluated at their own work station. If this is not possible, a computer work station in the clinic can be used. While working at the computer, the worker's posture, forces, and joint positions are evaluated. Document work pace, work station layout, and work-rest cycle (Keller et al., 1998). Videotaping the worker performing computer tasks allows for reevaluation. These tapes can be used to educate the worker in injury-prevention techniques and principles.

Table 6–1. Anatomical location, awkward posture, and potential diagnosis for computer users (Keller et al., 1998).

Anatomical Location	Awkward Posture	Diagnosis
Hand	Finger extension Thumb abduction	De Quervain's disease and trigger finger
Wrist	Ulnar deviation, hyperflexion, or extension	Guyon's canal syndrome, carpal tunnel syndrome, flexor carpi ulnaris, or extensor carpi ulnaris tenosynovitis
Forearm	Pronation	Intersection syndrome, pronator syndrome, anterior or posterior interosseous nerve syndrome
Elbow	> 90° flexion	Radial tunnel syndrome and cubital tunnel syndrome
Shoulder	Adduction, anterior humeral head, internal rotation	Cubital tunnel syndrome, medial and lateral epicondylitis, bicep contraction, thoracic outlet syndrome, and bicep tendinitis
Scapula	Protracted, elevated, winging inferior angle	Acromial impingement and suprascapular nerve entrapment
Neck	Anterior displacement	Anterior and middle scalene syndrome, cervical radiculopathy, and degenerative joint disease
Head	Forward	Temporomandibular joint dysfunction, headaches, and eye strain

RISK RESOLUTION/REDUCTION FOR COMPUTER USERS

Following identification of CTD risks, a systematic approach for risk resolution is recommended. Appendix F contains a sample ergonomic consultation report for a computer user. Hansford and Reiner (1995) encourage attention to the following when attempting to restore health and maintain well-being for computer users.

1. Corrective exercise

2. Biomechanically supportive work-station design

3. Functional keystrokes and input device usage

4. Balanced work habits

Extensive computer related, so-called "ergonomic" equipment is available, including chairs, pens, arm and wrist supports, and computer exercise stretch programs. Resources for some of this equipment are listed in Appendix A. Computer-related equipment should be recommended/purchased with caution (Claiborne & Williams, 1998). This equipment can be very costly and may not assist with resolving the underlying CTD risk factor. Often, currently available work stations can be adjusted/modified, and workers can be instructed in proper posturing and pacing principles for CTD resolution/prevention.

Keller and colleagues (1998) offer the following suggestions for CTD risk resolution:

■ Light key touching—relaxation and biofeedback techniques may be helpful; instruct the worker to press keys rather than lift and strike.

■ Use of biofeedback to assist with posture retraining (e.g., place electrodes on forearm flexors and extensors to provide feedback on cocontraction). Proper training in biofeedback is needed before this procedure can be performed.

■ A walking program to offset the sedentary nature of the work.

■ Splints to be worn only while sleeping and during retraining exercises.

■ Use of a rolling ball (smooth writing) pen with a built-up handle.

■ Pacing of activities—activity rotation, stretch breaks (program the computer to signal rest breaks), and relaxation techniques.

For workers who share computer workstations (e.g., several shifts), work-station adjustability is key. One size does not fit all. There is a lot of variability among workers including height, weight, health, and vision (Bello & Greenberg, 1998).

Work-Station Setup

A thorough review of computer work-station setup is out of the scope of this book. This section covers basic computer work-station setup recommendations as proposed by the American National Standards Institute (ANSI) (Bello & Greenberg, 1998).

Work-station chairs should be adjusted high enough to allow for straight wrists and elbows bent at 90°. A foot rest may be needed to place knees at 90 to 95° of flexion (Keller et al., 1998). The chair seat should be tilted to allow for 100° of hip flexion. The lumbar support should be adjusted between L1 and L5. Armrests should be equal to hip width with elbows at 90°.

The computer monitor should be placed directly in front of the worker, an arm's length away. The height of the monitor screen should be level with the top of the worker's head.

Documents should be placed in a document holder at eye level. Alternating the side to which the document holder is placed daily is recommended.

Work areas should be organized to minimize reach requirements. Materials used frequently should be located no more than a forearm's length away. Materials used occasionally should require only upper and lower arm reach. Infrequently used materials should require getting up and reaching forward or to the side.

The mouse should be at the same height as the computer keyboard. When using the mouse, workers' upper arms should be at their side with their elbows at 90°. If possible, alternate sides daily.

CHAPTER 7

Summary

The increased incidence of cumulative trauma disorders has led to an increased demand for injury-prevention services. An increasing number of occupational therapists are providing ergonomic services. The field of ergonomics provides occupational therapists with many opportunities. The occupational therapist can work in a variety of settings with a multidisciplinary team (Jacobs, 1993). Occupational therapists have a rich, work-based theoretical background that uniquely qualifies them for this setting. These unique qualifications include an emphasis on achieving independence in occupational performance with a holistic approach (ability to deal with physical and psychosocial issues). Specific occupational therapy skills that are helpful when providing ergonomic services include observation, activity analysis, and adaptive methods. Many of the ergonomic services occupational therapists are providing include risk analysis, ergonomic education sessions, and individual worker services (job analysis, job coaching, and worker education sessions).

This manual was developed to provide occupational therapists and students interested in providing ergonomic services with a basic ergonomic instructional manual and reference book. The purpose of this manual is to provide interested occupational therapists and students a basic overview of ergonomics and cumulative trauma disorders (CTDs), establish the theoretical role of the occupational therapist in this setting, and offer general practice guidelines for a variety of occupational therapy-based ergonomic services. This manual was developed as an introductory manual. Since this is a specialized occupational therapy area, additional reading and attendance at conferences are recommended to increase one's knowledge base and skill. A significant amount of ergonomic and CTD information is available from other professions (e.g., engineers, industrial hygienists, business people, and safety engineers). Several ergonomic and CTD conferences are also offered. Many of these conferences and courses are offered through University Industrial Hygiene and/or Ergonomic Departments. Conference listings in the occupational therapy literature also include ergonomic-related conferences.

Since very little occupational-therapy–specific research and literature related to CTDs and ergonomics is available, more publications and research would be beneficial. Occupational therapists have a lot to offer to the field of ergonomics including our functional approach and medical background. Additional research and publications will validate the role of the occupational therapist in the field of ergonomics and as a member of the ergonomic team. Research also is needed to demonstrate the benefits of occupational-therapy–based ergonomic services. Increased awareness of occupational therapists' contributions in this area and documented proof of the benefits of occupational-therapy–based ergonomic services will generate increased opportunities for occupational therapists in this specialty area.

APPENDIX A

Resources

REFERENCE BOOKS

Astrand, I. (1986). *Textbook of work physiology* (3rd ed.). New York: McGraw-Hill.

Chaffin, D. B., & Anderson, G. B. J. (1991). *Occupational biomechanics* (2nd ed.). New York: John Wiley.

Dul, J., & Weerdmeester, B. (1991). *Ergonomics for beginners: A quick reference guide.* London: Taylor & Francis.

Eastman Kodak Company. (1993). *Ergonomics design for people at work* (Vols. 1 & 2). Belmont, CA: Lifetime Learning.

Fraser, T. M. (1980). *Ergonomic principles in the design of hand tools.* (Occupational Safety and Health Series 44). Geneva: International Labor Office.

Grandjean, E. (1988). *Fitting the task to the man: A textbook of occupational ergonomics.* New York: Taylor and Francis.

Greenberg, L., & Chaffin, D. B. (1977). *Workers and their tools.* Midland, MI: Pendell.

Isernhagen, S. J. (1992). *Industrial physical therapy: Orthopaedic physical therapy clinics of North America.* Philadelphia: W. B. Saunders.

Isernhagen, S. J. (1992). *Work injury: Management and prevention.* Gaithersburg, MD: Aspen.

Isernhagen, S. J. (1995). *The comprehensive guide to work injury management.* Gaithersburg, MD: Aspen.

Macleod, D., Jacobs, P., & Larson, N. (1990). *The ergonomic manual.* Minneapolis: Ergotech.

Millender, L., Louis, D., & Simmons, B. (1992). *Occupational disorders of the upper extremity.* New York: Churchill Livingstone.

Murrell, K. F. H. (1965). *Ergonomics: Man in his working environment.* London: Chapman & Hall.

Pheasant, S. (1991). *Ergonomics, work and health.* Gaithersburg, MD: Aspen.

Putz-Anderson, V. (1988). *Cumulative trauma disorders: A manual for musculoskeletal diseases of the upper limb.* New York: Taylor and Francis.

Rice, V. (1998). *Ergonomics in health care and rehabilitation.* Boston: Butterworth-Heinemann.

Rowe, M. L. (1985). *Orthopaedic problems at work.* Fairport, NY: Perinton Press.

Salvendy, G. (Ed). (1987). *Handbook of human factors. Part 7: Designing for health and safety.* New York: John Wiley.

Sanders, M. S., & McCormick, E. J. (1987). *Human factors in engineering and design* (6th ed.). New York: McGraw-Hill.

Tichauer, E. R. (1997). *The biomechanical basis of ergonomics: Anatomy applied to the design of work situations.* New York: Wiley Interscience.

U.S. Department of Labor. (1991). *Dictionary of occupational titles* (4th. ed.). Indianapolis: JIST Works.

Wilson, J. R., & Corlett, E. N. (Eds.). (1990). *Evaluation of human work.* London: Taylor & Francis.

Office Ergonomic Books

Grandjean, E. (1987). *Ergonomics in computerized offices.* Philadelphia: Taylor & Francis.

Hansford, T., & Reiner, M. (1995). *Computer biomechanics illustrated.* St. Paul: Minnesota Hand Rehabilitation.

Mayfield, M., & Voge, L. (1989). *Computer comfort.* Mountainview, CA: Mayfield.

Salvendy, G. (Ed.). (1984). *Human-computer interaction.* Amsterdam: Elsevier Science.

INTERNET WEB SITES

General

Bad human factors designs, *http://gate.cruzio.com/~darnell/.*
Center for Industrial Ergonomics, *http://www.louisville.edu/speed/ergonomics/.*
Cornell Ergonomics Web, *http://ergo.human.cornell.edu/.*

Ergonomic Science, *http://ergosci.com/resources.html*. Educational site provided by the CTD resource network.

ErgoWeb, *http://www.ergoweb.com.*

Saf-T-Gard International, *http://www.saftgard.com/*. Safety equipment catalogs.

Office Ergonomic Web Sites

ACM/SIGCHI special interest group on computer-human interaction, *http://www.acm.org/sigchi/*. Equipment with EMG biofeedback.

Ergonomic Accessories and Furniture, *http:/www.workspace-resources.com/1ergo6.htm*. Ergonomic accessories and seating resource.

Ergonomic and Repetitive Strain Injury Lab Assessment, *http://www.sharetherapy.com/labassess.html*. Evaluation of ergonomic office.

Ergonomic Products, *http://www.tealresearch.com/tealproducts.html*.

Ergonomic Resources, Inc, GSA Resources, *http://www.ergonomicresources.com/gsa.html*. Ergonomic seating and work stations.

Grahl Ergonomic Office Seating and Chairs, *http://www.grahl.com/*.

Office Ergonomics, *URL:http://www.ur-net.com/office-ergo/*. Handouts for training sessions in office ergonomics.

Office Ergonomics Research Committee, *www.oerc.org.*

OSHA, *www.osha.gov.* Contains statistics and ergonomic guideline status.

Ergonomic Association Web Sites

The Ergonomic Society, *http://www-hcs.derby.ac.uk/ergonomics/*.

Human Factors and Ergonomics Society, *http://hfes.org.*

International Ergonomics Association, *http://www.louisville.edu/speed/ergonomics/international-ergonomics-association.html*.

Exercise Software

Ergodyne Worksmart Stretch Software: A fitness program for computer users. Provides simple stretching exercises that can be done right at the computer. (800)-642-5852.

CONFERENCES

Ergonomic Principles and Case Studies. University of Michigan Center for Occupational Health and Safety Engineering. (734) 763–0133.

Ergonomics and Injury Management Training Course, sponsored by Isernhagen & Associates. Isernhagen Work Systems, 1015 E. Superior St., Duluth, MN 55802. (218) 728–6455.

Ergonomics and More: Partnering with Business & Industry. Sponsored by Advanced Rehabilitation Services. (770) 973–3466.

Keith Blankenship. P.O. Box 5084, Macon, GA 31208. (912) 746–3792.

The National Ergonomics Conference and Expo. (212) 370–5005.

Systematic Approach to Industrial Rehabilitation. Matheson, L., 1160 North Gilbert St., Anaheim, CA 92801. (714) 491–1900.

Educational Handouts and Videos

CLMI Educational Videos. (800) 533–2767.

Krames Communication. (800) 333–3032.

Safety Clipart. P.O. Box 160932, Austin, TX 78716. (800) 767–8003.

JOURNALS AND PERIODICALS

Advance for OTs, PTs, and Managers. (610) 265–7812.
Journal of Hand Surgery. (800) 453–4351.
Journal of Hand Therapy. (215) 546–7293.
Rehabilitation Management. (310) 306–2206.
Work Injury Management. (913) 438–8400.
Work Journal: A Journal of Prevention, Assessment, and Rehabilitation. (212) 633–3730.

ASSOCIATIONS

American Occupational Therapy Association (AOTA). (407) 425–6011. Has a work special interest
    group.
American Society for Surgery of the Hand. (303) 771–9236.
American Society of Hand Therapy (ASHT). (816) 444–3500.
State Occupational Therapy Associations.

ERGONOMIC PROGRAMS

Isernhagen Work Systems. 1015 E. Superior St., Duluth, MN 55802. (218) 728–6455.
University of Michigan Center for Occupational Health and Safety. 1205 Beal, 154 IOE Building,
    Ann Arbor, MI 48109. (734) 763–4523.

ERGONOMIC CERTIFICATION

Board of Certification in Professional Ergonomics. P.O. Box 2811, Bellingham, WA 98227. (360)
    671–7601.

Sample Risk Analysis Report

The following is a portion of a risk analysis sample report. This analysis was performed at a small parts assembly plant. This plant assembles automobile seat control motors. The purpose of the risk analysis was to identify ergonomic risks and make recommendations for eliminating or reducing these identified risk factors. Table B–1 identifies ergonomic risks for various departments and offers recommendations. The data were collected through observation of the workers performing job tasks and interviews regarding job demands and physical stresses.

Table B–1. Small parts assembly risk analysis.

Job Title	Risk	Recommendation
Lid lock solder assembler	Forward head posture	Instruct worker to perform task with an upright, neutral head posture; issue worker an adjustable chair with sufficient upper and lower back support
	End-range wrist flexion when reaching into small plastic bin to retrieve connectors	Tilt the plastic bin forward to decrease wrist flexion when retrieving part
	Contact pressure both forearms (volar surface) due to sharp edge of work table	Pad edge of work station
Lever, spring and cover housing assembly	Contact pressure side of thumb and index finger as evidenced by workers taping fingers	Round sharp edges of plastic housing by designing a new injection mold for part; issue slip-on gel finger protection sleeves; lubricate part to reduce the amount of force required to assemble part
Connector and wedge insertion	High-pitched noise from small press when it cycles	Wear ear plugs
	Recessed finger buttons that require a significant amount of finger force and flexed wrists to depress	Replace finger buttons with soft touch palm buttons; relocate palm buttons to either side of press allowing for neutral forearm, wrist, and elbow position
Pump assembler	Forward head posture due to poor lighting	Replace lights with more sufficient lighting
	Worker stands on a concrete floor	Provide shock absorbent floor mats
	Contact pressure volar forearm when worker leans arm against sharp upright edge of conveyor	Remove sharp upright edge of conveyor; pad conveyor edge
	Use of very small hand-held clippers	Issue spring loaded clippers with padded and longer handles
Lid lock final tester	Vibration; excessive force and impact when pulling down lever of tester and holding while tester cycles	Lengthen lever to reduce amount of force required to pull and hold it; pad handle with shock-absorbant material or wear antivibratory gloves to reduce the effects of vibration and impact
	End-range elbow extension when reaching for tester controls	Relocate controls closer to operator allowing for neutral upper extremity positioning
Soldering position	Worker was observed holding small housing forcefully with left hand	Fabricate a jig to hold part while soldering

Note: In addition to the risks and recommendations listed here, the report would also include a brief job analysis for each job title and general plant ergonomic recommendations.

Ergonomic Educational and Training Handouts

The following five handouts reprinted in this section were designed by the Michigan Hand Rehabilitation center, Karen Williams, O.T.R., Director, and are reprinted with permission.

POSITIONS TO AVOID

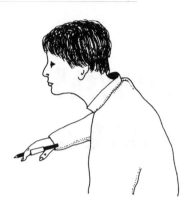

Forward head posture (head forward on spine)

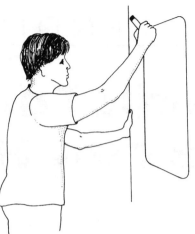

Reaching over the shoulder

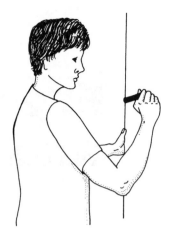

Elbow bent more than 90° angle (right angle)

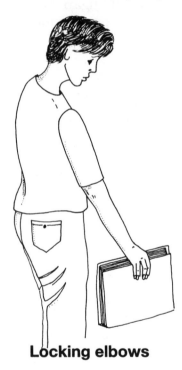

Locking elbows

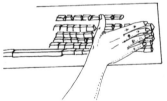

Radial deviation (wrist bent toward thumb)

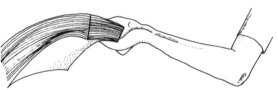

Flexion

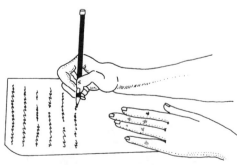

Ulnar deviation (wrist bent toward pinkey)

Supination-palm-up ESP-Hyperextension

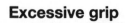

Excessive grip

Pinch with pressure

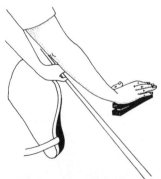

Pressure on the base of the palm

Constriction at wrist

ANTI-FATIGUE STRETCHING

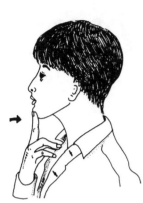

Chin Tuck

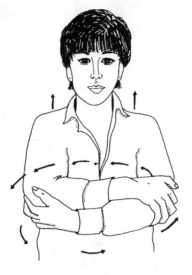

Relaxation Response #1

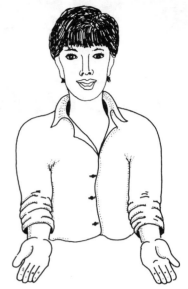

Relaxation Response #2

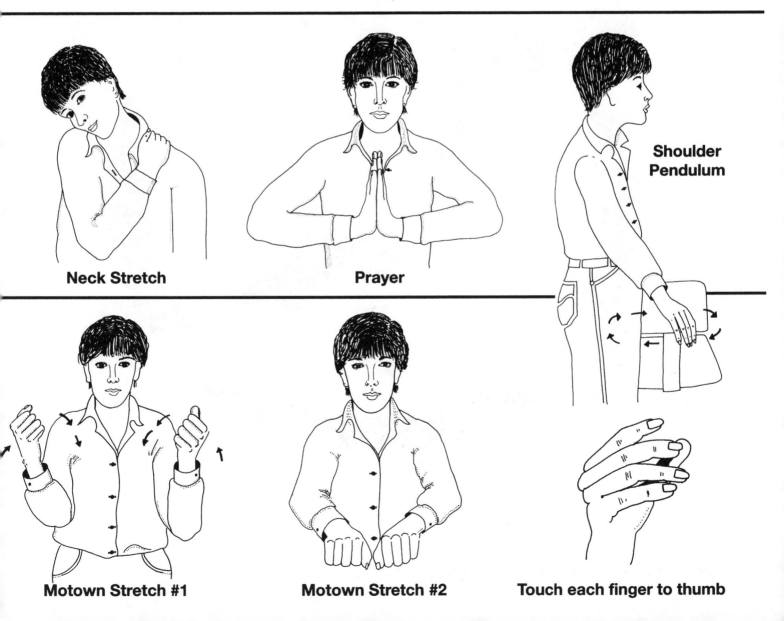

Neck Stretch

Prayer

Shoulder Pendulum

Motown Stretch #1

Motown Stretch #2

Touch each finger to thumb

FIGHT THE FIVE
Avoid These Postures

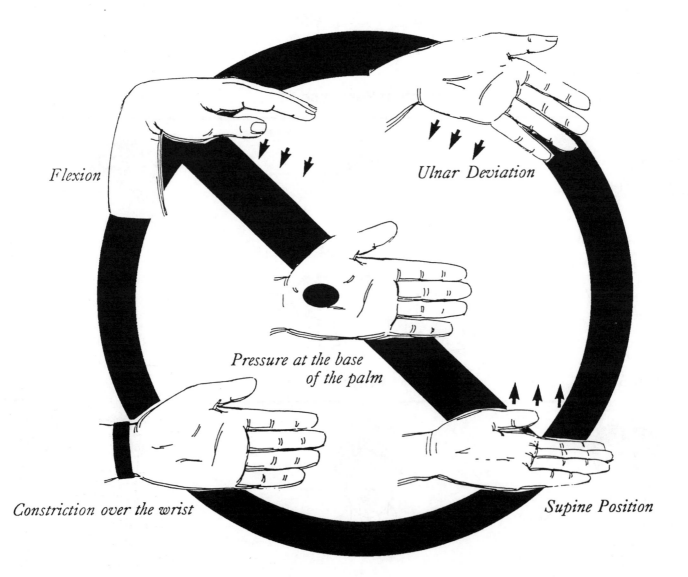

Flexion

Ulnar Deviation

Pressure at the base of the palm

Constriction over the wrist

Supine Position

Work Smart

Pace Yourself

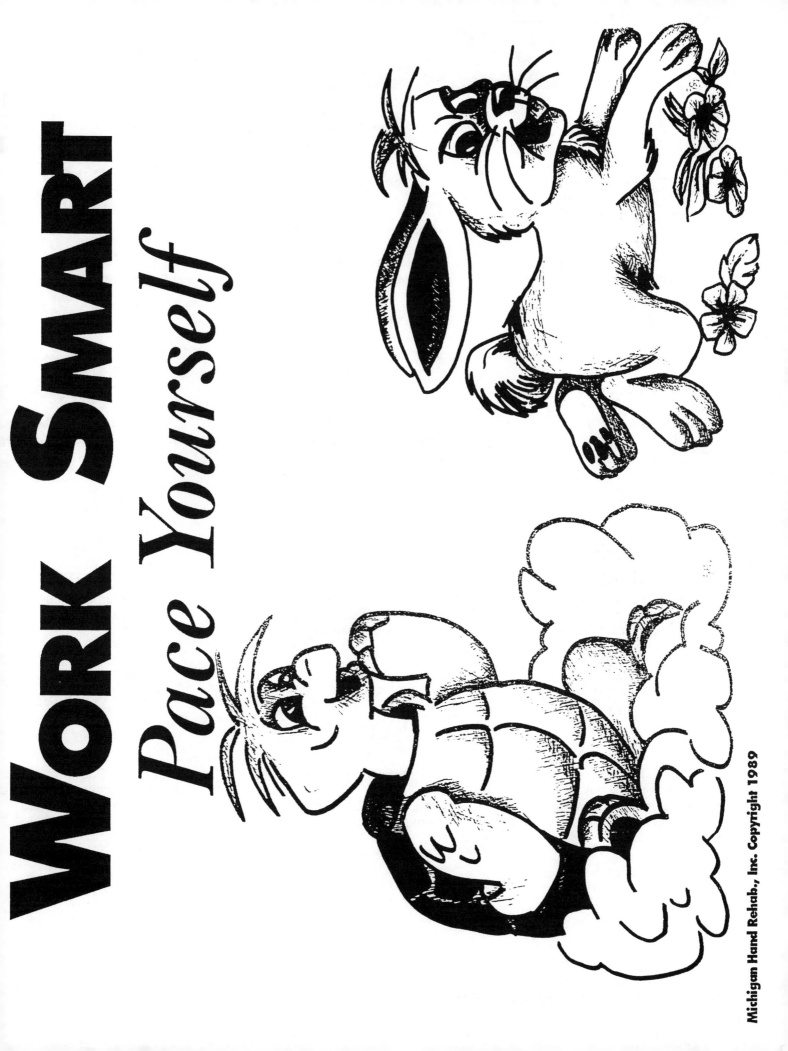

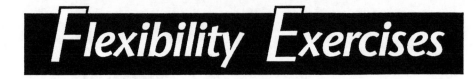

Flexibility Exercises

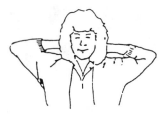

Reach behind your head
with both hands.

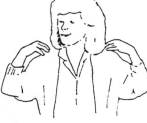

Touch both shoulders
with both hands.

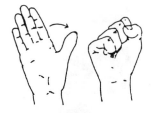

Gently open and close
fingers with wrist straight.

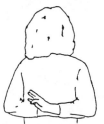

Reach behind your back
with both hands.

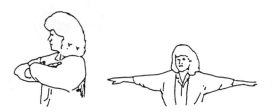

Cross arms at chest and
then stretch arms out at side.

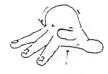

With palm flat on table, lift
each finger individually and tap

Neck Rolls
Start with chin down and
roll head clockwise and
then counter clockwise.

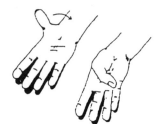

Hitchiker Thumb
Start with thumb out & then sweep
thumb across palm of hand
to base of small finger.

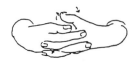

Twiddling Thumbs
Move thumbs gently in a
circular motion.

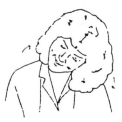

Side to Side
Bend neck towards your
right shoulder, then towards left,
hold on each side.

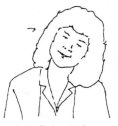

With your elbows at your
side turn palms up and then down.

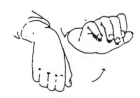

Wrist bends
Bend wrist down and then up
keeping fingers relaxed.

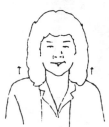

Shoulder Shrugs
Raise shoulders up and then down.

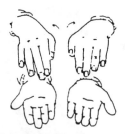

Wrist circles
Move wrist in a gentle,
smooth circular motion.

Make "O's"
Bring thumb to each finger.

Specialized Work Assessment Sample Report

Client: Sue Smith

Analyst: Jill Johnson, OTR

Employer: Lamps Are Us

Job Title: Lamp wirer

Contact Person: Ed Brown

INTRODUCTION

A specialized work assessment was performed January 9, 1997, at Lamps Are Us. The purpose of this assessment was to determine the physical demands of Ms. Smith's position as a wirer, identify any ergonomic risks, particularly as they related to her diagnosis of left-thumb De Quervain's disease, and make recommendations to reduce or eliminate these risk factors to assist Ms. Smith with returning to work.

Ms. Smith has a history of left-thumb De Quervain's. She has been off work and collecting worker's compensation for the past 16 months. Her medical treatment for this injury has consisted of two cortisone injections, a cast for 3 weeks, and 6 weeks of hand therapy that concluded December 23, 1997.

Workers typically work 8 hours a day, 5 days a week. Overtime is rare and is voluntary. Mr. Brown indicated that a graded return-to-work schedule beginning the middle of the week is possible. He reported rotation of positions is not possible since all positions have very similar job demands. He also commented that no restricted work (e.g., one-handed work) is available.

Workers were observed working at waist-high work benches on two-person teams. Mr. Brown indicated that if Ms. Smith had difficulty performing a few job tasks, her partner may be available to help her with completion of job tasks.

Mr. Brown indicated that there are no production requirements for this position. Workers were observed working at a slow steady pace.

Job Task Description

Equipment Used

Lamp base, cord, wire cutters, needle nose pliers, touch unit, crimping pliers, electric screw gun, adhesive felt, light bulb, plug cover, plastic bag, staple gun, and cardboard inserts

Physical Demands

Setup

1. Worker retrieved two lamps from conveyor and carried one in each hand 10 feet to the work bench. Lamp bases weigh 3 to 9 pounds. The lamps were stacked on the conveyor from floor to waist level. She repeated this process five times, filling the work bench up with a row of 10 lamp bases.

2. Worker retrieved 10 lamp cords located in a box on the edge of the work bench. She walked along the edge of the work bench, laying a cord next to each lamp.

Wiring

1. Worker trimmed cord ends with wire cutters (cut with right and held cord with left) and twisted wire ends with left hand.

2. Threaded cord up bottom of lamp base and out the top. She held the lamp in a gross grasp with left hand while threading with her right hand. Pulled wire through top of lamp with needle nose pliers held with right hand.

3. Spread wire apart approximately 2 inches, holding an end in each hand with a lateral pinch.

4. Inserted right and left wire ends into light base grooves, pressing in place moderately with both thumbs.

5. Sniped wire ends with wire snips while holding wire in place with left thumb.

Touch Unit Assembly

1. Inserted touch unit into light base groove. Held unit in place with left hand while crimping ends of unit with right.

2. Drove in one small central screw with right hand held screw gun. Screwdriver was located at eye level hanging from a retractable system.

3. Peeled off backing from adhesive felt and stuck to bottom of lamp base.

Testing

1. Tested lamp by screwing in a light bulb with right hand, while stabilizing lamp with left hand and plugging lamp in with right hand.

2. Snapped on lock cover with right hand while stabilizing lamp with right.

Packing

1. Held plug in a lateral pinch with left hand while putting on plug cover with right.

2. Lay plug in lamp saddle with right hand.

3. Pulled clear plastic bag over lamp, holding ends of bag in each hand.

4. Carried one lamp bilaterally over to finished lamp conveyor (approximately 5 feet) and placed on conveyor at ankle level.

Lamp Variations

1. Some lamps required a cardboard insert for packing. This insert was folded around the base of the lamp with both hands. It was then held in place with the left while stapled with the right using a hand-held manual staple gun.

2. Some (20 percent) of the lamps required a U-L knot. This consisted of spreading the wire approximately 4 inches, holding one end in each hand in a lateral pinch. The wire was then tied in a U-L knot, inserted into the bottom of the shell, and the cap was snapped in place with right hand. Approximately 50 percent of the lamps that required a U-L knot called for the gold cord. The gold cord was thicker and required significantly more force to pinch and pull apart than the brown cord.

Risks	Recommendations
Pinching and twisting wire ends with left hand	Twist ends with noninvolved right hand or alternate hands.
Holding wire ends in each hand with a lateral pinch while spreading wire apart	Develop a tool or use pliers with an angled handle in each hand to pull wire apart. This will decrease excessive pinch force requirements.
Pressing wire into light base grooves with thumb	Develop a tool that can be held with a gross grasp and neutral wrist position to press wire into place.
Contact pressure base of palm when using small, short-handled pliers and wire snips	Supply worker with longer handled tools that have lightly padded handles to spread pressure evenly across the palm.
Observed worker performing several tasks (e.g., threading cord into lamb base and using electric screw gun) with end-range wrist motions	Encourage and coach worker to perform these tasks with neutral wrist positions.
Excessive pinch force required to pull gold cord apart when making a U-L knot	Since this is a marginal job duty (only 10% of the lamps require the gold cord), it is recommended Ms. Smith not perform this job task.

General Recommendations

■ Trial return to work on a graded schedule. A suggested return-to-work schedule is as follows:

1. First week, 2-hour work days, 5-day work week
2. Second week, 4-hour work days
3. Third week, 6-hour work days
4. Fourth week, full 8-hour work days

■ Job coaching on return to work to encourage upper extremity wellness in the work place

■ Use of rubber grip gloves to increase grip ability while performing job tasks

■ Use fingers or tool to hold wire in place rather than thumb

SPECIALIZED WORK ASSESSMENT*

Name: _____

Date: _____

Employer: _____   Analyst: _____

Job Title: _____   Contact Person: _____

Patient #:

Introduction

A Specialized Work Assessment was performed on (date) _____

at (company) _____ to determine if (Mr./Ms.) _____

is able to meet the physical demands as a (job) _____ with respect

to (his/her) diagnosis of (diagnosis) _____ .

(Mr./Ms.) is currently (therapy, job status, etc) _____

_____

_____ .

At this time, workers typically work an _____ hour day _____ days per week.

(Hours are flexible upon return to work) _____

_____

_____ .

Rotations of jobs are _____ .

With respect to (Mr./Ms.) _____'s previous position, the

worker has the following physical demands (general for all jobs):

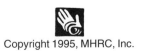

Specialized Work Assessment

Name: _____

Date: _____

Page 2

Job Task Description

Job Title:

Equipment Used:

Physical Demands:

Primary Motions of the Upper Extremity that are of Concern regarding (Mr./Ms.)

_____ :

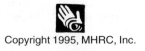

Specialized Work Assessment

Name: _____

Date: _____

Page 3

Job Title:

Equipment Used:

Physical Demands:

Primary Motions of the Upper Extremity that are of Concern regarding (Mr./Ms.)

_____ :

Specialized Work Assessment

Name: _____

Date: _____

Page 4

Job Title:

Equipment Used:

Physical Demands:

Primary Motions of the Upper Extremity that are of Concern regarding (Mr./Ms.)

_____ :

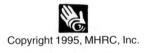

Specialized Work Assessment

Name: _____

Date: _____

Page 5

Summary/Recommendations

When comparing (Mr./Ms.) _____'s performance in (the work conditioning program, therapy program, FCE) at Michigan Hand Rehabilitation Center, Inc. with the physical demands of her job the following was noted:

Based on the above findings the following is recommended:

If you have any questions regarding this report, please do not hesitate to contact me at _____.

Respectfully,

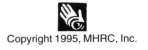

Job Coaching
Sample Report

Client: William Blank

Analyst: Jill Johnson, OTR

Employer: Baker Box

Job Title: Wrapper

Contact Person: Ray Blair

INTRODUCTION

An on-site job coaching assessment was performed on August 12, 1998, for Mr. Blank. Mr. Blank is presently working as a wrapper at Baker Box. Mr. Blank attended an individual worker education session at Hand Therapy, Inc., July 18, 1998. The focus of this education session was to teach Mr. Blank injury-prevention and pain-management techniques and principles. Mr. Blank is diagnosed with right lateral epicondylitis. Mr. Blank complained of frequent burning pain in the right lateral epicondyle. Mr. Blank has worked at this position for 2 years prior to this job coach. Mr. Blank was not working with any assistive equipment (e.g., splints or braces) during this job coach.

At this time workers typically work 8 hours daily, 5 days per week, with a 30-minute lunch break and two 15-minute breaks.

JOB TASK DESCRIPTION

Equipment Used

Box bottom inserts, wrapping paper and dispenser, tape and dispenser, and a pallet

Physical Demands

1. Worker retrieved approximately 50 box bottoms (approximately 36 pounds total weight) from pallet (stacked from ankle level to waist level) directly to his right and placed them on work table in front of him. The worker compared box bottom stack with a presorted stack to be sure there was the same amount in each stack. If the amount in his stack differed from the presorted stack, he adjusted his stack to match.

2. Worker tore a sheet of wrapping from dispenser located on work table to the worker's left. He then lay the paper on the table and smoothed it out.

3. Worker placed stack of box bottoms on the paper, wrapped the paper around the stack, and secured it with tape.

4. The worker pulled a short lever to dispense the tape and repeatedly tapped a water dispenser lever to wet the tape. The tape dispenser was located at the extreme right-hand corner of the table.

5. Worker smoothed tape on wrapped stack.

6. Worker lifted and carried wrapped stack and placed it on pallet located 4 feet behind him. The stacks were layered on the pallet from ankle level to shoulder level.

RECOMMENDATIONS

1. Encouraged Mr. Blank to lift one half a stack of box bottoms (18 pounds) at a time to decrease the weight lifted, and therefore decrease the strain on the elbow.

2. Instructed Mr. Blank in proper lifting techniques for back protection while picking up and lowering stacks. Retrieving and placing stacks in a squatted position will allow for midrange elbow postures.

3. Relocated paper to the center of the table to eliminate end-range right upper extremity reaching across midline to reach for and tear paper.

4. Instructed Mr. Blank to walk backward a few steps with elbows in a neutral position to unroll and tear paper rather than pulling paper with elbows fully extended.

5. Instructed Mr. Blank to turn stack when wrapping and tapping rather than reaching over stack.

6. Relocated the tape dispenser closer to the worker (to his right) and advised him to step to the dispenser rather then reaching for it with elbows fully extended.

7. Instructed Mr. Blank in simple neck, back, and upper extremity range-of-motion exercises to be performed prior to beginning work and whenever possible throughout the day to stretch and alter upper extremity positioning.

8. Encouraged Mr. Blank to use a cold pack for his elbow during lunch and breaks as needed for symptom relief.

ON-SITE JOB COACH REPORT SHELL*

Name: _____

Date: _____

Employer: _____   Analyst: _____

Job Title: _____   Contact Person: _____

An On-Site Job Coaching Assessment was performed on (date) _____

for (Mr./Ms.) _____ .

(Mr./Ms.) _____ is presently working as (job title) _____

_____

at employer) _____ .

(Mr./Ms.) _____ attended (a work conditioning, therapy, FCE)

_____

at (MHRC, Inc, or other) from (date began) _____ to (date ended) _____

regarding (diagnosis) _____

_____ .

He/She returned to work on (date) _____ , and is currently performing

_____

_____

_____ .

(Mr./Ms.) _____ is working with (assistive equipment, gloves, etc)

_____

_____ .

The purpose of these (assistive equipment, gloves, etc) _____

_____ .

On-Site Job Coaching Assessment

Name: _____

Date: _____

Page 2

 At this time, workers typically work an _____ hour day _____ days per week.

(Hours are flexible upon return to work) _____

_____

_____ .

Rotations of jobs are _____ .

 The following are the reported observations of (Mr./Ms.) _____'s

job coaching:

Job Title:

Equipment Used:

Physical Demands:

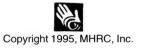

On-Site Job Coaching Assessment

Name: _____

Date: _____

Page 3

Client Concerns:

Client Successes:

Recommendations:

If you have any questions regarding this report, please do not hesitate to contact me at _____ .

Respectfully,

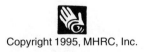

Ergonomic Consultation Report for a Computer User

Employer: Software USA

Job Title: Software Engineer

Analyst: Joan Smith, OTR

Client: Theresa Brown

Date: May 7, 1998

An on-site ergonomic consultation was performed May 7, 1998 for Ms. Brown. She is currently working as a software engineer. Ms Brown has received extensive treatment for her bilateral arm, neck, and shoulder symptoms including therapy, acupuncture, and several on-site ergonomic assessments from various providers. She has been previously issued extensive ergonomic equipment, including computer and mouse tray, ergonomic chair, various mouse operating systems, phone headset, document holder, foot rest, and voice-activated dictation system. Despite treatment and issued equipment, Ms. Brown continues to complain of neck, shoulder, and arm symptoms.

Ms. Brown reported her current symptoms include burning pain in her thumbs which radiates up to her elbows and stabbing pain with spasms in her upper back and bilateral shoulders.

Ms. Brown was instructed in antifatigue exercises and posture do's and don't's. She was also instructed in the use of cold packs at home and work (during breaks) for symptom management.

Clinical Observation

Ms. Brown was noted to have forward head posture, forward rolled shoulders, and wrist hyperflexion and ulnar deviation while working on the computer. She required moderate reminders to maintain neutral postures during the remainder of the job coach.

Job Task

Computer keying

Equipment Used

High back chair, foot rest, computer, mouse, keyboard tray, desk

Observed Risk	Resolution/Recommendation
Poor posture while seated at the computer	Adjust chair back forward and upright, tilt seat slightly backward, and adjust lumbar insert to between L1 and L5.
Forward head posture when looking at monitor	Slide monitor forward on desk to within arm's length to reduce eyestrain and improve head, neck, and shoulder posture.
Elbows >90°	Lower chair to allow for 90° elbow flexion.
Static upper extremity posturing due to lack of arm support	Adjust arm rests to hip width and allowed for 90° elbow flexion.
Ulnar deviation when using mouse and keyboard	Slide her forearms using larger shoulder muscles rather than wrist deviators.

References

American National Standards Institute (ANSI). (1996). Draft-Z-365. *Control of work related cumulative trauma disorders, Part 1: Upper extremities.* Washington, DC: Government Printing Office.

Armstrong, T. (1994, June). *Analysis and design of jobs for control of upper limb musculoskeletal disorders.* Paper presented at The University of Michigan Occupational Ergonomics Conference, Ann Arbor, MI.

Baxter-Petralia, P.L. (1990). Therapist's management of carpal tunnel syndrome. In J. M. Hunter, L. H. Schneider, E. J. Mackin, & A. D. Callahan (Eds.), *Rehabilitation of the hand: Surgery and therapy* (3rd ed.). St. Louis: Mosby.

Beattie, M. C. (1995). Determinants of lumbar disc degeneration. A study relating life time exposure and MRI findings in identical twins. *Spine, 20,* 2601–2612.

Bello, R., & Greenberg, S. (1998). *Office ergonomics.* Paper presented at Ergonomic and Injury Management Training Course, Philadelphia, PA.

Bettendorf, R. F. (1998). A framework for understanding upper extremity musculoskeletal disorders. A paper from The Office of Ergonomic Research Committee Inc. [On-line]. Http://www.oerc.org.

Bureau of Labor Statistics. (1994). *Survey of occupational injury and illness by selected characteristics.* Pub. No. USDL 94–213. Washington, DC: Author.

Butler, D. (1998). Ergonomics and Injury Management Training Course. Sponsored by Isernhagen Work Systems, Philadelphia, PA.

Cannon, N. M. (1991). *Diagnosis and treatment manual for physicians and therapists* (3rd ed.). Indianapolis: The Hand Rehabilitation Center of Indiana, P.C.

Chong, I. (1993). Ergonomic solutions stop the "loop" encountered in worker's compensation costs. *Occupational Health and Safety, 7,* 31–32, 53.

Claiborne. D. K., & Williams, K. (1998). Cost-effective ergonomics. *OT Practice, 3,* 47–48.

Devlin, P. (1993). Briefs. *Work Injury Management, 2,* 16–17.

Dunn, W. (1988). Models of occupational therapy service provision in the school system. *American Journal of Occupational Therapy, 42,* 718–723.

Dutton, R. (1993). Rehabilitation frame of referance. In H. Hopkins & H. Smith (Eds.), *Willard and Spackman's occupational therapy* (8th ed.). Philadelphia: J. B. Lippincott.

Framroze, A. (1994). Does ergonomics fit your career path? *Rehabilitation Management, 7,* 37–40, 43.

Grandjean, E. (1988). *Fitting the task to the man: A textbook of occupational ergonomics.* New York: Taylor and Francis.

Harms, J. (1996). *Selling physical therapy and industrial rehabilitation services in the worker's compensation market presentation.* Sponsored by Work Injury Management News & Digest, Managed Health Resources, & Advantage Health Systems, Atlanta, GA.

Hansford, T., & Reiner, M. (1995). *Computer biomechanics.* Duluth, MN: Minnesota Hand Rehabilitation.

Imker, F. W. (1993). What constitutes an ergonomics program. *Work Injury Management, 2,* 8–11.

Isernhagen, D. (1998). Ergonomics and Injury Management Training Course. Sponsored by Isernhagen Work Systems, Philadelphia, PA.

Isernhagen, S. J. (1988). *Work injury: Management and prevention.* Gaithersburg, MD: Aspen.

Isernhagen, S. J., Hart, D. L., & Matheson, L. N. (1998). Rehabilitation ergonomists: Standards for development. *Work: A Journal of Prevention, Assessment, and Rehabilitation, 10,* 199–204.

Isernhagen, S. J. (1998). Ergonomics and Injury Management Training Course. Sponsored by Isernhagen Work Systems, Philadelphia, PA.

LaBar, G. (1991). Bent out of shape. *Occupational Hazards, 53,* 37–39.

Jacobs, K. (1985). *Work related programs and assessments.* Boston: Little, Brown.

Jacobs, K. (1989). Use of the Department of Labor references and job analysis. In S. Hertfelder & C. Gwin (Eds.), *Work in progress: Occupational therapy in work programs.* Rockville, MD: AOTA.

Jacobs, K. (1993). Work assessments and programing. In H. Hopkins, & H. Smith (Eds.), *Willard and Spackman's occupational therapy* (8th ed.). Philadelphia: J. B. Lippincott.

Johnson, K. (1993). Wellness programs. In H. Hopkins & H. Smith (Eds.), *Willard and Spackman's occupational therapy* (8th ed.). Philadelphia: J. B. Lippincott.

Kasdan, M. L. (1991). *Occupational hand and upper extremity injury and disease.* Philadelphia: Hanley & Belfus.

Keller, K., Corbett, J., & Nichols, D. (1998). Repetitive strain injury in computer keyboard users: Pathomechanics and treatment principles in individual and group prevention. *Journal of Hand Therapy, 11,* 9–25.

Kenny, D., Powell, N. J., & Reynolds-Lynch, K. (1995). Trends in industrial rehabilitation: Ergonomics and cumulative trauma disorders. *Work: A Journal of Prevention, Assessment and Rehabilitation, 5,* 133–142.

Kirkpatrick, W. (1990). Dequervain's disease. In J. M. Hunter, L. H. Schnieder, E. J. Mackin, & A. D. Callahan (Eds.), *Rehabilitation of the hand: Surgery and therapy* (3rd ed.). St. Louis: Mosby.

Kroemer, K. H. (1989). Cumulative trauma disorders: Their recognition and ergonomic measures to avoid them. *Applied Ergonomics, 20,* 274–280.

Matheson, L. N., Ogden, L. D., Violette, K., & Schultz, K. (1985). Work hardening: Occupational therapy in industrial rehabilitation. *American Journal of Occupational Therapy, 39,* 314–321.

Mayer, T. G., & Gatchel, R. J. (1988). *Functional restoration for spinal disorders: The sports medicine approach.* Philadelphia: Lee & Febiger.

Moore, H. R. (1990). OSHA: What's ahead for the 1990's. *Personnel, 67,* 66–69.

Nathan, P. A. (1990). Work related carpal tunnel syndrome. *JAMA, 263,* 236–237.

Pelletier, K. R. (1993). A review and analysis of the health and cost effective outcome studies of comprehensive health promotion and disease prevention programs at the work site: 1991–1993 Update. *American Journal of Health Promotion, 8,* 50–62.

Pheasant, S. (1991). *Ergonomics, work and health.* Gaithersburg, MD: Aspen.

Putz-Anderson, V. (1988). *Cumulative trauma disorders: A manual for musculoskeletal diseases of the upper limbs.* New York: Taylor and Francis.

Rice, V. J., & Jacobs, K. (1993). Ergonomics, you're legitimate. *Rehabilitation Management, 4,* 39–43.

Rice, V. J. (1998). Certification in ergonomics. *OT Practice, 3,* 25–30.

Taylor, S.E. (1993). Industrial rehabilitation. In H. Hopkins & H. Smith (Eds.), *Willard and Spackman's occupational therapy* (8th ed.). Philadelphia: J. B. Lippincott.

Trombly, C. A. (1989). *Occupational therapy for physical dysfunction* (3rd ed.) Baltimore: Williams & Wilkins.

Ulin, S. (1997). Ergonomic principles and case studies conference. Sponsored by The University of Michigan Center for Occupational Health and Safety Engineering, The Safety Council of West Michigan, and The Public Health Consortium, Grand Rapids, MI.

Weber, L. J., & Karen, L. A. (1998). OSHAs proposed ergonomic standards: Impacts and outcomes. *Work: A Journal of Prevention, Assessment, & Rehabilitation 10,* 31–39.

Werner, R. (1997). Ergonomic principles and case studies conference. Sponsored by The University of Michigan Center for Occupational Health and Safety Engineering, The Safety Council of West Michigan, and The Public Health Consortium, Grand Rapids, MI.

Whitenack, S. H., Hunter, J. M., Jaeger, S. H., & Read, R. L. (1990). Thoracic outlet syndrome complex: Diagnosis and treatment. In J. M. Hunter, L. H. Schnieder, E.J. Mackin, & A. D. Callahan (Eds.), *Rehabilitation of the hand: Surgery and therapy* (3rd ed.). St. Louis: Mosby.

Index

DATE DUE

SEP 26 2005			